Managing Difficult Patients

A Guide for Nurses and Other Health Workers

Richard Miller, RMN, BA, Dip.N.Ed.

D1477341

ff

faber and faber

LONDON · BOSTON

First published in 1990
by Faber and Faber Limited
3 Queen Square London WC1N 3AU

Photoset by Parker Typesetting Service Leicester
Printed in Great Britain by
Cox & Wyman Ltd Reading Berkshire

A CIP record for this book is
available from the British Library.

ISBN 0-571-14127-7

Contents

Figures

ACKNOWLEDGEMENTS

I would like to thank the staff and students I have worked with over a number of years who have helped me in formulating many of the ideas in this book, and acknowledge that much of this work is a description of current good nursing practice. I would especially like to thank my wife Meg for her help and encouragement. This book is dedicated to Mr Stanley Holder OBE, FRCN for his contribution to nurse education and for providing an environment in which I could develop many ideas and skills.

Introduction

This book is about how to manage aggressive patients and it seems to me that there are four possible reasons for reading it:

- to learn to avoid trouble
- to learn to write good nursing care plans
- to learn self-defence
- to learn how to be a better nurse.

Those reading this book for the first three reasons will be disappointed. Furthermore, they are not yet ready to nurse the aggressive patient if they want a 'cook-book' of action to take when confronted with aggression. In this area of nursing the way the nurse does things and why are as important as what she does. Being a successful manager of aggression is more about being something than it is about doing something.

While the nursing process and individual care planning are what distinguishes nursing from the allied professions this is not a book about care plans – except that it might be about an individual plan for the nurse. Those wishing to know more about care plans are referred to Collister (1988).

There is no attempt to teach self-defence in this book. Anyone wishing to learn to defend themselves should attend a class run by a qualified person. It even avoids the teach yourself approach in the area it deals with, in order not to create in the reader that false sense of security this approach gives rise to. Instead, it provides ideas and information the nurse can use to help her acquire the skills she needs in fulfilling responsibility, meeting trouble and surviving. It is an introduction to the cognitive (thinking) and affective (emotional) aspects of managing difficult patients.

Some of the views expressed are not in keeping with more traditional approaches and it may be that some nurses will find parts of the book provocative. The aim is not to be provocative for its own sake, but to raise relevant issues for the reader to think about. Thinking is an important part of learning and a skill that should never fall into disuse.

There are no formulae for action offered of the sort that say 'If you do this then no one will hit you.' This book is about how the nurse can develop herself to be more able to manage the aggressive patient. What is central to the effective management of aggression is skill in interacting with other people. This is so important that the ideas described in Chapter 4 derived from Transactional Analysis might be seen as a model of all nursing, not just aggression management.

There are a number of important points underlying the effective management of aggression. Knowing these might help the reader to understand the general approach of this book.

(a) Most aggressive incidents would be prevented if intervention were to take place at the time when the person begins to be difficult.

(b) All of us, no matter who or what we are, can be difficult. Difficult behaviour arises from the individual's perceptions of the situation and personality and role make a major contribution here.

(c) The way to reduce the occurrence of difficult behaviour is to be adult. Occasionally the nurse can use the positive 'child' and the positive 'parent' positions (see Chapter 4).

(d) The nurse must actively manage the difficult patient by using the adult qualities of clear communication, good stress management, self-awareness and respect, empathy and genuineness.

(e) When prevention fails and aggression and violence occur the nurse must act in a deliberate manner to contain the situation.

(f) Education and training are central to the development of the skills needed to be an effective manager of aggression.

These ideas have not been scientifically established, although there is much research to support the reasoning behind them. (There is a shortage of research in this area.)

There is no substitute for experience and so only by being

confronted by aggression can the nurse become skilled at managing it. However, training and education are indispensable to prepare the nurse for such experiences and modern methods of nurse education are ideal. Only through education can the nurse develop the personal qualities which will help her to avoid provoking aggression and aggravating the aggressive patient. And she can develop the behavioural, affective and cognitive skills she needs only by being prepared to expose herself to methods of personal development.

Chapter 1 deals with personality and role. It aims to emphasize the importance of individual differences and the idea that while most people have little control over their personality it is possible to develop aspects of it.

Chapter 2 presents a view of 'social skills' and their relevance to the nurse. Chapter 3 continues this theme by looking at self-awareness, an essential component in developing social skills and in helping the individual to shape her own personality.

Chapter 4 contains the central message of the book, that in order to reduce the likelihood of aggressive incidents the nurse should behave in an 'adult' manner when interacting with other people.

Chapter 5 discusses why the nurse might find another person's behaviour difficult and presents five ways in which someone can be difficult. Chapter 6 presents a summary of how these forms of difficult behaviour might be dealt with.

The idea that the way the environment is presented to the patient can be a major contributor to difficult behaviour is discussed in Chapter 7. Of course it is also true that this is one way of reducing difficult behaviour. Chapter 8 applies the same approach to the individual nurse. It offers suggestions about how she might become more adult in her presentation and thereby reducing to a minimum her contribution to difficult interactions.

The psychological approaches to preventing difficult behaviour sometimes fail and the individual becomes aggressive or violent. The nurse needs then to utilize physical measures to manage the situation. These are discussed in Chapter 9. Chapter 10 deals with the way a policy might be formulated to help staff manage aggression. The nurse's responsibility is discussed in the final chapter.

1 Personality and Role

PERSONALITY

The study of personality is important for nurses as it can provide guidance both when developing policies and procedures and in their practice (Davis 1981). A knowledge of personality and its development will help the nurse to a better understanding of others and of the differences between herself, her colleagues and her patients. By having knowledge of the way in which individuals have grown to be different she will find it very much easier to tolerate and to enjoy those differences. It is then easier for her to take account of the great variety of human behaviour. It is important for the nurse who finds herself confronted by a difficult patient to understand how the patient has come to be in that state. She will be more able to help him to become cooperative and to take his needs into account. Of course, by understanding her own personality and her own role, she will be more able to predict her own behaviour and fulfil her own needs.

Some aspects of personality have an effect on physical health. Many characteristics of personality have popularly been associated with poor physical health, but while many of these beliefs have not stood up to scientific scrutiny there are some that do (Wood 1988). For instance, it is predictable that some personality qualitics will be associated with illness or accident. Those who are more careless than most can expect to have more accidents. Someone with a negative view of themselves is more likely to become saddened and depressed.

Knowledge of personality may help the nurse to plan care and to understand others. For example, recent work has shown that people who tend to be more alert in the evening are better able to function during the night than those who are more alert during the morning.

A senior nurse may view one nurse as being competent and motivated and another as careless and disinterested, yet the real difference between them may be in the way they respond to night duty. That response is biological and generally beyond the control of the individual. Around four in the morning is statistically a high risk time for accidents and an 'evening person' is less likely to make mistakes during the early hours.

Personality is the sum of all the individual's qualities which are evident in behaviour and taken together make the individual unique. It is the sum of individual differences. Most of these qualities arise as part of normal healthy development. While they have a tendency to be consistent and enduring they are generally open to modification.

Theories of Personality

There are many theories of personality and its development. Many of these overlap and there seems to be no useful way of categorizing them. Freudian theory, for example, includes biological, social and learning components and is concerned primarily with unconscious processes. Skinnerian behaviour theory is traditionally seen as contrary to Freudian ideas but includes both biological and learning components. As its name implies it is concerned with observable behaviour and claims that underlying processes are irrelevant. The two approaches represent the extremes of personality theory and most other theories are derived from or associated with one approach or the other.

There is no single theory which accounts for the depth and complexity of human personality. Many theories give a good account of some aspect of personality but not one is both comprehensive and general. Freudian theory can be unrealistic, restrictive, subjective and can present a very pessimistic view of humanity. Behaviourism is very specific and objective but tends to make an irrelevance of the individual's feelings. While they are without doubt useful in helping to conceptualize some pathological conditions and their treatment, these theories are limited as theories of normal personality and development.

Trait Theories

To overcome some of the difficulties associated with studying personality, each theorist has tended to look at a limited area of personality. Problems have then arisen when the creator or the users of a theory have treated it as a general theory. One approach which has taken a more sophisticated view of personality is that of traits. The trait approach looks at separate traits or groups of traits which tend to occur together while accepting that the individual has many others which are not being considered. There are over four thousand words available in the English language to describe traits. Even if we reduce the number of traits an individual can have to as little as one hundred, and even if we count them only as being present or not present there exists the possibility of millions of millions of unique individuals. Since the four thousand traits are mostly present in varying degrees in all of us, there is an almost infinite variety of human potential.

Examples of Traits   Traits include such things as extroversion, introversion, prejudice, tolerance, aggression, passivity, attitudes towards authority, morality, maturity, stability and creativity.

Creativity is a good example (Vernon 1970). It is strictly speaking a group of traits (Guilford 1970) and is associated with such traits as tolerance of ambiguity, divergent thinking and flexibility (Reazik 1970). A creative person has these and other traits in greater quantity than a less creative person. Such traits as divergent thinking may themselves be made up of or influenced by other traits working together.

A quality such as divergency is important to nurses (Adams 1987; Jones 1983). Divergent thinkers are more productive in creating new ideas and new ways of doing things and are possibly less defensive and rigid. Yet they are less accepted and accommodated by education systems (Parnes 1970) and other organizations. Indeed 'organization' and 'divergency' are sometimes contradictory. There may be conflict when an organization demands conformity from a divergent thinker. It is also difficult for those who are fundamentally convergent and those who are fundamentally divergent to understand each other, since a convergent thinker tends to prefer things to remain the same while a divergent thinker tends to prefer continuing change.

A divergent thinker is less well organized than a convergent thinker, who is able to apply far more structure to her activities. The structure makes a converger and her work much more comprehensible to most other people and may mean that she gets more work done.

A divergent thinker is less likely to be judged as performing well in an organization, like the health service, say, and is therefore less appreciated and less rewarded. The constraints of the system are more likely to be unacceptable to her and she will therefore seek satisfaction in outside interests such as hobbies and sports activities. She may also develop other interest associated with her work by taking a greater interest in academia or developing a speciality. Alternatively she may leave and seek satisfaction in less structured employment.

Convergent thinkers stay longer in jobs and tend to do well in hierarchical bureaucracy, and are more likely to be rewarded there (Adams 1987). In the extreme, convergers will be rigid, authoritarian and afraid of change, while divergers will be totally disorganized, unable to concentrate and disruptive. Fortunately very few people are totally convergent or divergent and everyone has a mixture of both traits in varying quantities.

Calling someone convergent or divergent implies no judgement of them. It is an observation of what is probably a genetic and perhaps biological tendency over which the individual has little control. Society needs both kinds of thought – divergent for invention and exploration and convergent to provide stability and continuity.

Another important trait is that known as 'hardy personality' (Kabosa, Kahn and Maddi 1982). An individual who has the qualities which contribute to this feels that she has a large degree of control over life and her experience of it, she believes in what she does and sees difficulties as a challenge. She is therefore less prone to stress and anxiety and more able to cope with it when it does occur (Geer and Maisel 1972; Seligman 1975; Seligman *et al.*

1979). Because of this she can lead a more fulfilling life and is more likely to achieve her goals. She has better mental health than a 'non' hardy person.

Eclecticism One of the advantages of a trait approach to personality is that it offers a choice of areas to explore and where appropriate the ability to select the theoretical framework which is the most useful or productive for practice. In this way theory becomes something that can be used to develop practice rather than a template that restricts it. The most useful parts of different theories can be gathered together to provide the most suitable approach for a particular case. It is possible, for instance, to take a behavioural approach when treating a patient suffering from anorexia nervosa, this being the most useful in-patient treatment. However, where a wholly behavioural approach is adopted the patient may undergo little change. Good practice in the treatment of anorexia nervosa includes involving a third party (someone other than the ward team) to provide a more exploratory approach and to encourage personal growth and development.

Eclecticism uses those parts of any theory which are most appropriate to current needs. The choice will depend on the approach of the practitioner and the problem to be solved. The danger of eclecticism is that the choice of components is subjective. Audley (1967) concludes that people's minds are already made up and that only information which fits in with previous decisions will be accepted. This is evident in such people as politicians – both armchair and elected, doctors (Butler-Sloss 1988) and nurses. Decision-making will work best where there is a problem-solving approach and where there is a democratic style of management allowing issues to be discussed and explored (McFarlane 1976; McGregor 1960; Marriner 1980). An authoritarian management style will discourage divergency. This is an important element in effective problem-solving (Adams 1987), although convergency is also important as it will give more direction and structure to the problem-solving.

Nursing tends to take an eclectic approach (McFarlane 1976; Frost and Nunkoosing 1989). To the extent that a nurse strives for and uses problem-solving to enhance objectivity and recognizes the value of a democratic approach the difficulties associated with subjectivity and decision-making should be less of a problem. For an eclectic approach to personality see Bee (1989).

Personality Development

The question of nature versus nurture is one that frequently arises. Today few practitioners would claim that personality is solely a product of either hereditary or environmental factors. Research suggests that genetic factors shape basic personality or set the boundaries in which development takes place according to the environment encountered and the way the individual interacts with it (Mussen *et al.* 1969).

However, any factors which can be reliably identified in personality are likely to arise from a mixture of influences. In most cases the interaction between environment and genes will be such that it becomes almost impossible to describe single influences. It is of course impossible in most cases to distinguish the effects of 'nature' from 'nurture' when exploring the behaviour of real people. Additionally the degree to which knowledge can be structured is limited by lack of knowledge. Very little is known about what happens in the brain and the mind.

Mussen *et al.* (1969) bring some structure to this debate. In a fairly comprehensive work they identify five categories of influence on the developing personality: genetically determined, non-genetic biological, past learning, immediate social psychological environment and the general social and cultural variables. Because of the interaction of influences and the complexity of behaviour it becomes difficult to distinguish between these categories. The only universal in personality development is the passage of time and it is important to remember that personality development is lifelong. Many of the psychological skills are associated with the development of personality and many normal and ordinary experiences throughout life make a contribution to this. Figure 1.1 illustrates the development of personality.

Figure 1.1 The development of personality

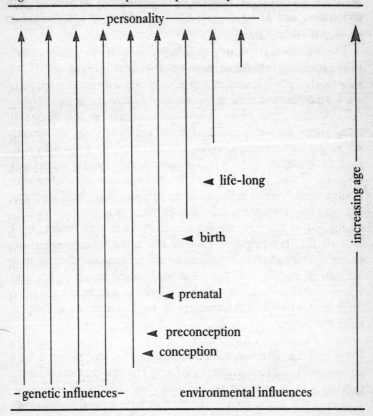

personality

◄ life-long

◄ birth

◄ prenatal

◄ preconception

◄ conception

increasing age

–genetic influences–   environmental influences

Genetic Factors Generally speaking the genetic variables are those qualities we inherit from our parents, few of which are modifiable. They include, for instance, eye colour, nose shape, skin pigmentation, hair colour and type, overall body shape and size, intensity of physical reaction to anxiety, blood pressure, age of onset of menstruation and longevity.

There is no doubt that these physical characteristics can influence personality. Height, weight and skin colour all affect how a person interacts with the environment thereby helping to shape personality. Even a quality like nose shape may affect confidence and therefore development. However a large, small or indifferent nose will only be one of many influences on personality. A nose cannot account for personality.

The boundaries of some psychological variables have been shown to be genetically influenced, mostly by the use of twin studies. These variables include IQ, tendency to introversion/extroversion, responses to strangers and tendency to smile. All these can be modified as the individual grows older and continues to develop. It is likely that many other normal personality traits are genetically influenced. There are also abnormal variables, such as those associated with Down's Syndrome and PKU. It is quite possible and in some cases quite likely that abnormal genetic variations are associated with environmental factors acting upon the parents. After birth influences are primarily environmental although there may be some genetic disorders that affect personality which do not become evident until later in life, Huntington's Chorea and acute schizophrenia, for example. Some genetically influenced normal variables also may only become evident in later life – eventual weight range, height and sexual characteristics, for example. All this can make it even more difficult to know if influences are to be described as genetic or environmental.

Pre-birth Environmental Influences   The environment does not only affect the person after he is born. The embryo and the foetus develop in the environment of the womb and are affected by it.

During the period from conception to birth a number of factors might influence personality (Haddad 1985). If the mother drinks too much or smokes it will affect the child. Other influences at this time could be mechanical or chemical – drugs, some foodstuffs, level of nutrition, radiation, metal poisoning and anoxia, for example. It is also possible for the foetus to learn; it can be conditioned, albeit in a simple way, and may learn such things as anxiety from its mother.

Birth Influences   The most obvious influence at birth is that associated with a difficult birth. This itself may be genetically influenced, the mother having inherited certain characteristics from her mother or her father, hip size, for example. There may also be cultural influences. For example, one way of inducing anoxia in neo-nate experimental monkeys is to hold the placenta below the newly arrived monkey so that the blood flows away from the monkey depriving it of oxygen. The effect, however marginal, of prone delivery and other modern practices on the 'average' IQ and other abilities of the population is not known.

Life-long Influences The environmental influences which act on us throughout life are experience (which includes learning), maturation (including growing and ageing), physical experience (which includes trauma, illness, recovery from illness and such things as keep-fit and body-building).

Learning is a life-long process. The new-born infant is able to learn at a rapid rate where there are no barriers to prevent it (isolation from stimulation and anoxia, for example). This rate of learning potential decreases with age as the individual leaves childhood and grows older, but with increasing age people develop more sophisticated learning skills and become more deliberate in their learning.

An important part of experience is those people who are close. These are normally parents, siblings and peers. All have an influence on growth and development. Workers such as Bowlby (1984) and Harlow (1971) have described this. As well as influencing by example and direction they are also the people on whom children (and to a lesser extent adults) practise interactions. Later in life new behaviour is developed in relationships with spouse and offspring. The lessons learnt from the important people in early life are put into practice on almost everybody encountered.

Other social factors have been demonstrated by Asch (1952), Bandura (1977), Bryan and Test (1967) and Milgram (1974). These may be less direct than some of the others but are still very important. They can become especially evident at times of conflict. This can be seen in reactions to the Falklands War, at times of civil unrest and in the tribal behaviour (Morris and Marsh 1988) of football supporters.

People are not passive in their development. Response and

reactions to the environment and to other human beings within it help to shape future development. A person interacts with the environment and future personality is influenced by present environment.

What is quite clear is that it can very rarely be said that a particular piece of behaviour is a direct result of a particular influence. The influences described above are not explanations of behaviour but principles underlying the development of the personality, which is the major influence on behaviour. They cannot offer a definite explanation of someone's actions, thoughts or feelings but should help to develop an understanding of why people do the things they do.

ROLE

One of the ways of deciding how to interact with others is by considering roles (Cox 1983). A role is a set or series of behaviours associated with a particular position in a society or group. Roles are shaped by the expectations of those occupying the role and of the relevant people associated with that role. These expectations prescribe the appropriate behaviour of the roleholder.

Role therefore varies across time, place and person. The role of England's monarchy over several centuries is a good example of this. Sometimes the expectations of the monarchy have been comparatively subtle, as perhaps at the present time when the monarch has been able to determine her own style. At other times those expectations have been more overt, as for instance during the English Civil War of 1642–5 when Cromwell and the parliamentarians very forcibly expressed their expectations of the monarchy and therefore changed its role.

Over time and at any one time we occupy many roles, such as father, husband, son, charge nurse, bus passenger, shopper, footballer, etc. Sometimes roles occur in sets such as father, husband and brother-in-law. Roles may be in conflict as when a charge nurse is admitted as a patient. They are rarely isolated from each other as many of them interact, and they all interact with the role-holder's personality.

Some roles are transient, such as that of student, child and passenger. Some, like being male or female, are permanent although some of the roles associated with being male or female may not be. At times it is unclear when a role ends. Wing-commanders, majors and doctors all retire but retain their title and many of the qualities associated with the role. It is hard to decide to what extent some roles, that of son for instance, diminish with age and if they stop when for instance the father dies. Will I still feel like my father's son after he has died?

Some roles are thrust on us. Inescapable roles might include being a child or being male and some of those arise because of a pre-determined place in society – citizen, schoolboy and patient. Others are chosen – nurse, passenger and union member. Some of these chosen roles are actively sought and others are just accepted. What is a sought role for one person may be inescapable for another.

A charge nurse on duty is occupying a role. The expectations he has which shape his role are a result of his personality and his experiences (including his training). His role is also shaped by the patients, the staff and those close to him. Other more distant people also shape his role, the UKCC (UKCC 1984), the pay review body, the DHSS/DoH/DSS (DHSS 1989; DSS 1988) and politicians. While some of these seem powerful and distant they also are influenced by others. Such organizations are influenced by the people who serve in them, those who govern them and those who are governed by them.

A well-known but perhaps less well understood example is the 'sick role'. It is generally credited to the patient, being seen by many as a criticism. It is often used to describe an individual who 'wants to be sick' or at least does not wish to regain independence. But a patient adopting the sick role has an obligation to want to get better (Cox 1983) and so to want to be sick is a contradiction of the role's real meaning and the nurse often demonstrates a failure to under-stand the role.

It is the expectations of the patient, his relatives and of the staff which prescribe the patient's role. That will include the nurses, doctors and other care workers who must share some responsibility for the adoption and functioning of such a role. That responsibility may include failure to be influential enough to prevent the patient adopting the role. The misconception of the sick role is a good demonstration of the need to increase understanding and knowledge to help improve the performance of health workers.

There are people who adopt the sick role in order to prolong their time as patients. That they need to stay patients as long as possible has more to do with anxiety and fear, loneliness and lack of confidence than it has to do with 'the sick role'.

A patient may be occupying roles other than 'patient'. He remains a father, son or husband. He still has a bank account, an income and bills. He may also be adopting a role which influences his reactions to illness, hospitals and the staff. He may have come from a background in which his role models responded to illness by denying it in order to help maintain their dignity. This will cause him conflict when he needs care. It may be he learnt that part of the patient's role is to allow feelings of hostility or suspicion to come to the surface.

As a father I have experienced much frustration and anger when taking my child to our local Accident and Emergency (A&E) department. The staff have at times seemed unsympathetic and have kept us waiting for long periods. A parent anxious about his child's well-being will be more vulnerable and volatile than at other times. The role of parent makes additional demands on the individual. There are occasions when the role-holder may have difficulty in meeting the demands and expectations associated with that role, in this case ensuring a child's comfort and well-being. This situation is known as 'role strain' and can be very stressful.

SUMMARY

It is important for the nurse to have a knowledge of personality and role to help her understand the differences between herself and others. No one theory has accounted for the complexity of personality and the depth of feelings people experience. By being aware of the diversity of influences at work on personality the nurse will find it easier to tolerate difficult behaviour, which may be beyond the control of the patient. Influences can be described as either genetic or environmental, but while they can be so categorized it is difficult to identify specific effects. The individual's social behaviour is also influenced by his role. A role is determined by the expectations of the role-holder and those associated with that role. Readers wishing to know more about personality should refer to the general psychology texts available. The most comprehensive of these is Atkinson *et al.* (1983) (previously known as Hilgard and Atkinson). Those wishing to know more about role will find Cox's (1983) book useful.

2 Social Skills

An important part of the nurse's work is to interact with the patient. Where the nurse is skilled in her interactions the patient will have a greater understanding of the nurse's communication and therefore be more able to cooperate with her. This is true of all the nurse's interactions with the patient. It is especially important when the nurse is in contact with individuals who are particularly vulnerable or prone to aggressive and violent behaviour. An unskilled nurse will provoke difficult behaviour in otherwise reasonable people. The skills which a nurse can use to be an effective interactor are generally described as social skills. The absence of social skills in the nurse is one of the factors which will increase the incidence of difficult behaviour. A socially unskilled patient will experience more difficulties in coping with a system and those in it.

All nursing tasks are based on interacting with the patient or with someone else on the patient's behalf. Non-nursing tasks, such as clerical and portering tasks, are generally not interactionist. Many managerial tasks are not nursing. Filling in a time sheet for an organization which already has a record of the nurse's work is bureaucratic and is not related to patient care. It may be that bureaucracy arises as a substitute for interacting. Many of the functions of senior nurses relate to the functioning of the organization and not to patient care.

Because of its strong interactionist element nursing is a unique practice. While there is overlap with other professions no one else serves the same function as a nurse. It is sometimes hard to describe that function and some nurses have great difficult in being able to say what it is that they do which makes them special. Indeed this author has heard several nurses up to and including charge nurse grade state that good nursing is common sense. Common sense is exactly what good nursing is not. It may contain elements of good sense, but quite clearly good nursing practice is only achieved through education and experience. Indeed, it would seem that many components of good nursing are about overcoming 'common' sense.

As an example of a common sense approach a group of students described a 'doctor's ward round' in a psychiatric unit which claimed a multi-disciplinary approach. When the doctor wished to see the patient a nurse went to the patient and brought him to the meeting. The patient then sat in whichever chair had been left vacant, usually opposite the consultant and with the sun in his eyes, was asked questions first by the doctor and then by others. At no time was the patient asked if he knew everybody present or if he had any objections to them all being there and was not offered a chance to ask questions. This was a ward round conducted using common sense. There was little professional practice.

A professional ward round would have been called a team meeting and included such things as the patient being accompanied into the meeting by the person who has the best relationship with him; being allowed a choice of chairs and to sit next to someone he found supportive.

All staff should introduce themselves or remind the patient who and what they are and the patient should be given opportunity to request a smaller or different group of people to be present and the specific opportunity to ask questions. All this need not be stage-managed to any great degree. It should arise naturally from the staff having a positive view of themselves and others. If care is left to common sense then patients are not given the attention and care they are entitled to.

Other professional groups will be offended by the suggestion that they are not interactionist. Quite clearly doctors, psychologists and occupational therapists do interact, but the study of interaction is not the most important part of their science. Although doctors are expected to have a good bedside manner clearly many of them don't and it seems to be a part of nursing culture that the nurse is expected to compensate for the doctor's failing (Butler-Sloss 1988; Royal commission 1978), possibly because doctoring is a class-related profession which has a vested interest in political and personal power. Doctors behave as if they are powerful people with the authority to make decisions about other people. This may be acceptable to some patients but it causes many problems. They behave as if they alone know best and they seem to believe that the way they interact is not important to the patient. See, for example, Hamilton and Freeman (1982), Hardy (1985) and Priest and Wolfson (1978) for illustrations of the low value the medical profession has of interactional skills when compared with technical skills and knowledge.

It would be wrong to claim that all doctors are like this and that nurses never are. Some doctors are very good at interacting and some nurses are very bad (Hempel 1988). The difference is that the nursing profession is addressing this issue in a way that the medical profession is not. The way they interact is perhaps one of the most important issues for nurses, being central to the nursing process and to all new training initiatives and proposals. On the other hand, the main issue for medicine seems to be the level of science which is to be practised.

While professions like psychology and occupational therapy (OT) also have some interactionist elements the practitioners tend to be very selective about who they interact with and have narrower, often very specific, aims. Nurses are required to interact with anybody who needs their care and are not allowed to deny that care to any one for any reason which is not therapeutic (UKCC 1984). Furthermore that care, which includes the way the nurse interacts, must be delivered in a reasonably egalitarian way. Where others fail to interact appropriately the nurses, in their roles of communicator and advocate, are called upon to compensate (Butler-Sloss 1988; Royal Commission 1978). Nurses have an obligation to be, and are the people that others rely on to be, skilled interactionists.

Nurses need a wide range of interactional skills and are often called upon to switch rapidly from one kind of interaction to another. A nurse on a medical ward may have to interact with a confused old man; turning from his bed she may encounter a difficult and offensive teenager. She may have in adjacent beds a man of great intellect and one who is mentally handicapped. Her patients may include someone who is painfully compliant and someone who is unable to comply. The patients may be unconscious or active and they may wish to stay a patient forever or be desperate to leave the nurse's care. This cross-section of people contributes to the uniqueness of the nurse's role. For this and other reasons it is important that the nurse's interactional skills are especially well-developed (Niven 1989).

INTERACTIONAL SKILLS

In order to identify the interactional skills it is necessary to first consider the nature of interactions, the reasons for and benefits of interacting. A way of evaluating interactions would also be useful.

The Nature of Interactions

An interaction takes place when two or more people communicate in any way. It may be verbal or non-verbal, explicit or implicit, face-to-face or remotely (by telephone or perhaps by letter) and knowingly or unknowingly. Of course not all interactions are of equal quality. The ritualistic greetings exchanged by fellow commuters cannot be said to have the same value as those which pass between a nurse and a patient at the beginning of the shift. Nor is that nurse–patient greeting of the same value as that between a nurse and a close colleague. The way greetings are exchanged with loved ones is of a different nature to all of these.

It may be that greetings will be more important, with more effort involved, if there is some expected gain in the interaction. The something may be material, it may be associated with a service or may be targeted at an emotional gain such as recognition or warmth.

For the interaction to be effective there must be some element of mutual benefit, but not necessarily one that is material. For instance, it may be that some people just like being nice to others, or that they like people to be nice to them. And strange as it sounds, in the same way that some people find being nice a rewarding experience others may find being difficult rewarding.

It will be assumed here that there are two parties to any interaction, self and other(s). The environment is not included as a factor because the individual's reactions and responses to it are more important. This is not to say that the environment has no importance in psychology, sociology or nursing. Quite clearly it has. But it is perhaps easier to view the environment as a background against which interactions take place. Discussion of practical aspects of managing the environment is included later. Responses to the environment are an important part of an individual's make-up. They vary from person to person and from time to time.

If a description of interactions includes the surroundings as a part of that interaction a difficult problems presents itself. Are other people a part of the environment or do they enter an inter-action in their own right? The answer to this question will depend on the psychological and/or sociological beliefs of the respondent. There seems to be a continuum of opinion which ranges from seeing others as unimportant except as environmental features, to others being seen as an active influence in their own right. The place that any other person occupies on this continuum depends on the degree of their closeness or relatedness to you.

For a student nurse on the first day of her first ward most of the people on it seem like environmental features. More than anything she will be concerned about herself and what she is experiencing at a time of stress and anxiety. As she gets to know the ward (including the people) she will begin to differentiate between various aspects of it. She will identify the individual differences that each person possesses and will therefore be able to differenti-ate more easily between one person and another. The processes of getting to know people and of becoming closer to them are com-plementary. As the nurse gets to know someone she becomes closer to them and as she becomes closer to someone she finds out more about them. This is true at both a superficial level and at a more personal level. Of course, this is also true for the patient. A nurse who has been seen at a distance on another part of the ward has little individuality to a patient. If the patient then uses the nurse call system and that nurse arrives, she is seen as more of a person but perhaps not yet as an individual. After they spend some time together and perhaps share some activity the patient is able to identify the nurse's individuality and the nurse begins to interact as an individual rather than as a part of the environment.

For the purpose of this book it will be assumed that the interaction takes place between two (or more) people who have become significant in their own right.

Reasons for Interacting

Interactions have several purposes:

(a) To give instructions, information and advice.
(b) To receive instructions, information and advice.
(c) To help a patient solve problems.
(d) To improve mental health.
(e) To be polite and socially acceptable.
(f) To offer comfort and reassurance.

The first two of these are basic communication. There is a need to communicate in order to find out about the patient and his care. This communication takes place with the patient, relatives, other carers and colleagues. Basic (common) skills are not adequate for this task and the nurse needs to develop special skills.

A patient has been admitted for removal of, and tests on, a growth. The tests have shown that it was an early malignant tumour. The nurse approaches the patient and tells him that it was malignant but that it has been caught early and was therefore easily removed with little further risk. The patient is likely to be tense and to have difficulty in concentrating. He will hear the nurse tell him that the lump was malignant but is unlikely to hear or remember much else because of his thoughts and feelings about the first piece of information, that he has a malignant growth. He may not know what malignant means, but it's obviously bad news. Is he going to die? Will it be painful? What about his wife? Is the insurance valid? What is the nurse nattering about?

It is important for the nurse to have the skills to deliver the information in a way that allows the patient to receive it. It is the nurse's responsibility to be able to do this. It is not up to the patient to acquire high level communication skills in order to understand those who care for him.

The nurse needs to be able to gather information to aid her decision-making. She must pay enough attention to her patient to be aware that he is no longer listening to her and be able to recognize his emotional state by the way he behaves and the things he says.

A good example of the benefits of good communication is Hayward's (1975) work in which he was able to demonstrate that informed patients required less analgesia. Skilled communication also affects the validity of consent. A patient must have an understanding of what he is consenting to in order for the consent to be valid. 'Don't worry, old chap, it's just a little operation – nothing to worry about' is not enough. It must be informed consent. The patient may not need to *know* but must *understand* what is to happen to him.

Another aspect of nurse-patient interaction is providing comfort. It is likely that a comforted patient will be more cooperative, more able to understand and more able to help himself. All other things being equal his stay in hospital will be shorter, and therefore cheaper, if this comfort is provided. He will have a more positive view of hospitals and health care and be more likely to make good use of them in the future. He will be more willing to consult somebody at an earlier stage of an illness and to receive earlier and more effective care.

As a separate issue there is the patient's right to be comforted. There is no good reason why there should be any undue suffering in our society and especially in relation to health care. Suffering at some time or other is unavoidable for all of us and life can at times be very painful. It is a part of the nurse's role to help reduce the suffering of the painful parts of life and to help people to be able to enjoy the good parts. This can only be achieved through skilled personal contact with the patient.

Counselling is a form of interaction associated with good communication (Buckroyd 1987; Egan 1985; Nurse 1975; RCN 1978). Counselling is aimed at enabling a person to arrive at solutions to their own problems in their own ways in their own time. It is a facilitative process relying on high-level skills.

In much the same way as he or she needs the right physical activity to maintain physical health so a person also needs the right mental activity to maintain mental health (Fries and Crapo 1981). Social isolation leads to degeneration of social skills and is associated with many negative feelings, especially about self. By interacting with others a patient is able to maintain and improve his mental state. He is also able to test his anxieties and fears against the reality offered by other people. The patient's mental well-being will enable the nurse to deliver more effective care to him. As with comfort, everyone has the right to the best possible mental health.

It is reasonable to expect nurses to behave in an educated, civilized way, a component of which is the possession and demonstration of good manners. Nurses are professional members of society and should behave as such. Good manners are also bound up with good communication and other social skills. Life is generally easier and less stressful when people are polite to each other.

Skilled interactions will make the nurse's work more effective and therefore easier and more economical (Harris 1988; Niven 1989). The better the nurse's social skills the better her interactions will be. Normal healthy contact with other people helps keep patients (and nurses) mentally fit and healthy and makes life more bearable and enjoyable. Each person has the right to be treated in a reasonable and polite manner, especially people who are in need of care and support.

IDENTIFYING SOCIAL SKILLS

Because nursing is a social activity, nurses are required to possess what are generally described as 'social skills' (Hargie and McCarten 1986). The need is evident if the range of nursing functions are considered. Throughout her shift a nurse is constantly in contact with other people, many of whom rely on her for essential information, as a carrier of messages and as a guide through the system. The nurse must do all this in a constructive and encouraging way. As the nurse in charge of a department she is the central figure and the demands on her will be considerable. The more socially skilled she is the easier she will find her task and the more successful she will be in fulfilling her role.

Everybody possesses some social skills. Knowing who to say 'good morning' to and when to say it is a social skill. It is a low-level skill but can be developed and combined with others to produce high-level skills.

Most discussion of social skills associated with nursing relates to psychiatric nursing. They should in fact be regarded as core skills for all nurses, and not just part of good psychiatric nursing practice.

Many authors refer to social skills without specifying what they mean. For instance, in a useful work Pope (1986) is able to tell us what criteria might be applied to define social skills and what features they possess but does not include a comprehensive description of them. He does talk of the components of communication behaviour which might be included in social skills. This is similarly true of Argyle (1972), Barker and Frazer (1985), Dexter and Wash (1986) and French (1983), all of which are useful texts. Hargie and McCarten (1986) take a more specific approach than the other authors. They summarize several works when they describe social skills as being behaviour which is goal-directed, appropriate to the situation and which can be learned and is under the individual's control. They discuss these qualities at length helping to clarify the meaning of social skills by doing so. But this is itself does not make it easier to identify the specific social skills.

This lack of 'lists' of social skills has three causes: first, because rigid definition of social skills is a contradiction of the open-mindedness needed to possess them; second, human behaviour is so complex that it is very difficult to describe its components in a neat, ordered and structured way, and third, there seems to be no commonly agreed criteria for differentiating the variety of skills used by human beings (see, Burnard's (1989) view). This situation is in some ways desirable as it allows flexibility in dealing with social skills. The more general the description of these skills the greater the range of practical applications. However, knowing some of the qualities of social skills does not necessarily help to identify them or understand what to do with them. This makes it hard for the beginner and those only marginally interested to know what is going on.

Several of those authors already mentioned suggest that social skills are specific abilities which are needed to perform the everyday tasks associated with conversations, encounters and relationships, and Argyle (1972) describes them as the style of social behaviour used. These views do not include all social skills and a specialist approach (that of a therapeutic social skills training, for example) may only be useful in specific situations. For more general situations a more general approach is needed. It may therefore be best to look at social skills in several different ways.

PSYCHOLOGICAL DOMAINS

It is common practice in psychology to divide human functions into three categories, sometimes mistakenly called skills, attitudes and knowledge. These are correctly identified as *behaviour*, *affect* and *cognition* and are useful in considering social skills. The behavioural skills are those which are demonstrated in the actions of an individual. This includes all that can be seen and measured. The cognitive skills are those involved in thinking. They include such functions as decision-making, problem-solving, knowledge, reasoning and some aspects of perception. The affective skills are associated with feelings, their effect and their presentation. Attitudes and motivation are examples of affective components.

Self-control, for example, is probably an affective skill, but it has elements of cognitive skills – using reason and problem-solving to help contain emotions. It is also evident in a person's behaviour and must therefore have some behavioural components.

Because they have been concerned with practical skills most skill theories are behavioural in approach, but this need not be so. For example, there are well-identified affective and cognitive skills involved in decision-making (Adams 1987). Argyle (1972) sees social skills as having a number of components: they are social behaviour, are effective and are used to realize a goal. Some social skills, such as using a ticket machine or deciding what to buy for lunch, do not in themselves require any interpersonal behaviour.

A GENERIC APPROACH

It may be more useful to describe social skills as any mastered behaviour which enhances the individual's social functioning. The activities of daily living (Roper *et al.* 1983) include skills, that is they are learned and with practice become automatic. They can sometimes be carried out without any contact with other people, but they are often done because of other people and are very often a part of a life shared with others. They are most noticed when neglected. The failure to do such things as bathe, be presentable and to eat a balanced diet can be seen as anti-social. A failure to be acceptable will interfere with the individual's social activity. Bathing is therefore a social skill or perhaps a group of social skills. It is not however seen as such by most writers and many practitioners. Similarly the ability to make sense out of the world has a profound effect on our social behaviour but is only really noticed when there is a failure to be skilled.

If the term 'social skills' is used as a generic heading to include all skilled behaviour which effects our social activity we can then include a number of subheadings, which might include, for example:

- Interpersonal skills, which include the quality of our interactions and our understanding of others.
- Communication skills, such as talking, listening, reading, writing and non- and sub-verbal skills.
- Perceptual skills, such as perception and interpretation.
- Motor skills: coordination and the ability to move about in order to use other skills.
- Decision-making, which might include other cognitive functioning.
- Living skills, such as the activities of daily living and any other skills used to carry out the activities used to prepare for social interaction.

It would be nice to present this as a neat hierarchy of skills with each level contributing to the next. In reality these groups of skills are a network each contributing to every other and all dependent to some extent on all the others.

Identifying Specific Skills

Another way to look at social skills would be to try and identify them in their broadest presentation and to become increasingly specific in describing them. This is not suitable for a general introduction to social skills but let us consider communication as an example. Effective communication is not a single social skill but a product of many, and one component skill in it is non-verbal communication (Hargie 1986; Hargie and McCarten 1986). One form of non-verbal communication is eye contact (Argyle 1981; Rutter *et al.* 1981). A part of skilled eye contact is direction of gaze and specific use of gaze is to indicate turn in interaction (Harrigan and Steffan 1983). This could be further dissected to look at speed of movement, accuracy of direction, and so on. If this approach was adopted and taken to its extreme there would be so many identified skills that their simple description quickly becomes impossible.

A PROCESS APPROACH

An alternative approach could be to look at the social processes involved, at what will here be called the primary social skills and then at the secondary skills.

Social Processes

These include – personal interactions, social interactions and functional interactions.

Personal interactions are those involving others when they are important because of who they are. This will generally be with relatives, friends and colleagues but might include others who have not previously met but who have some special contact. An example of this might be a fellow passenger on a train.

Social interactions are with individuals who are not important in their own right. These might be shop assistants, other shoppers, people casually encountered at a party or workers from another department. Interactions with relatives and friends might sometimes be social rather then personal.

Functional interactions are of two types, those which serve geographical functions and those which serve mechanical functions. When a driver is using a road at the same time as someone else he must be aware of the other and respond in certain ways while obeying certain rules. The two drivers do not normally interact on a social or personal level. This kind of interaction takes place because people happen to be in the same place at the same time, it is geographical.

There are some social processes involving other people which are mechanical. They could be carried out by machines. Ticket collectors on the railways perform such a function. It is not normally necessary to have any social or personal contact with them. Most ticket collectors and passengers do not talk to or even look at each other. A machine could do the work just as well. Indeed, machines which do the work are now increasingly available.

To perform these interactions people need a number of primary and secondary skills:

Primary skills include observation (of others),
                         receiving communications,
                         sending communications,
                         self-presentation,
                         physical activity.

Secondary skills include activities of daily living,
                         activities in support of daily living,
                         other private activity,
                         cognitive skills,
                         affective skills.

Those social skills which are needed to take part in an interaction might be described as 'core' skills (Hargie and McCarten 1986) and are clearly related closely to communication skills. Indeed many nursing writers seem to equate social skills with communication skills. While this may at times be true it is a narrow view. There are occasions when an individual needs core skills which are not directly associated with communication.

Primary Skills

Those skills which are used when face-to-face with another can be described as being primary. The primary skills are those which are used during interactions, are mostly seen in behaviour and include the core skills. Interacting individuals observe each other and the situation in which they meet because they need to gather information to enable them to make decisions concerning the interaction. Communication can be verbal, sub-verbal (noises, affectations, etc. used in speech but which have no grammatical value) and non-verbal (body posture, facial expression, etc.). Self-presentation becomes a skill noticed by its absence. While some of these primary skills will be directly associated with communication others, such as dress sense, will for most of the time be independent. Physical activity includes those actions undertaken when interacting and which can be practised. These range from moving towards and away from someone in an appropriate way through to intimate sexual activity. Figure 2.1 is a list of a few examples of aspects of primary social skills. Most readers will be able to expand this list which is neither comprehensive nor definitive. Some items are very general some are more specific.

Figure 2.1 Some aspects of primary social skills

appropriateness of gaze	chronology of body contact
duration of gaze	level of intimacy
direction of gaze	speed of contact
placing of body	clarity of speech
direction of body	speed of speech
direction of movement	volume of speech
'uprightness' of posture	length of utterance
style of walking	facial expression
dress sense	eye contact
eating behaviour	inclination of head
drinking behaviour	position of arms, hands, trunk, etc.
duration of handshake	movement of arms, hands, trunk, etc.
strength of handshake	expression of deference
appropriateness of body contact	use of obscenities
strength of body contact	tutting, etc.

Secondary Skills

The secondary skills are those which enable an individual to use the primary skills. The activities of daily living (Roper *et al.* 1983) are clearly essential to the ability to use primary social skills. In order to perform the activities of daily living there are many other things that people need to do. In order to keep his hair clean a young man needs soap and water. To acquire shampoo he needs to visit a shop, which includes activities on the way to the shop, at the shop and on the way home. To get hot water he needs to notify the water and power supplier that he has taken over occupation of his residence and to pay the bills.

Some skills which effect daily social life might be quite private. Reading, for example, is not something generally shared with others. By reading an individual can gather information to be used socially. Reading may also act as a diversion allowing the individual to relax and to tolerate and enjoy social activity. A long hot bath or a hobby might have similar effects. Figure 2.2 lists some of the secondary social skills.

Figure 2.2   Some aspects of secondary social skills

maintaining a safe environment	use of a hobby
eating and drinking	ability to use household appliances
eliminating	sportsmanship
controlling body temperature	ability to sit still
self-expression	problem-solving
sleeping	decision-making
use of public transport	remembering
driving ability	knowing
parking ability	perceiving
personal mobility	understanding
letter writing	respecting
bill paying	loving
use of telephone	tolerance
cooking	flexibility
basic home care	optimism
domestic work	authority

It is important to remember that those listed in the figure are examples of areas of social skill. All the activities mentioned need to be appropriate to be skilled and sometimes doing something which is socially unacceptable can be skilful. Appropriate use of smiling is a social skill but so is the appropriate use of frowning. The lists are intended to help a newcomer to think about and to understand what is meant by social skills, especially when primary social skills are discussed. They are not intended as a guide to the use of social skills.

All the examples in Figure 2.1 will enhance the nurse's interactions. Many of those in Figure 2.2 should also be important to the nurse, enabling her to help her patients and making her own life more rewarding. Like all skills these can be learnt and developed. The process of skill acquisition is the collection and interpretation of information, deciding what needs to be done, action and feedback (Legge and Barber 1976). This is of course repetitive – the more times it occurs the better the skill. There are similarities between this process and problem-solving.

SUMMARY

A nurse should develop her social skills to enable her to function more effectively. If she is going to help her patients achieve more in their lives she has to understand and be able to describe and demonstrate the social skills. Additionally, and just as important if not more so, by becoming highly socially skilled the nurses's life will be enhanced. Specialist approaches take a narrow view of social skills but a more generic approach might be more useful for most nurses. The approach described suggests that many skills not traditionally seen as 'social' are involved in social activity and can therefore be described as being secondary. The primary social skills are those evident during interactions.

3 Self-awareness

FEEDBACK

Feedback is an essential component in skill acquisition (Legge and Barber 1976; Milne *et al.* 1985). This is true of both sensory-motor and social skills. When performing a task, knowledge of results is needed to achieve optimum performance. Any attempt to navigate is futile if decisions are not checked out against results in order to note progress or the lack of it. Travellers lost in the desert or forest who wander in circles have little or no feedback on the results of their attempts to find their way to safety. A successful typist does not observe the act of typing but looks at the results of it.

Receiving inaccurate feedback will initially contribute to a poorer performance than receiving no feedback. Consistently inaccurate feedback can be allowed for and with practice the individual can compensate for the inaccuracy. An example of this is the way experimental subjects respond when wearing spectacles which invert or offset the visual field (Stratton 1897). Initially they can feel nauseous and have great difficulty moving about but after a while they begin to behave as if their visual field was normal. They have adjusted their knowledge of the world and the feedback they receive about their performance in it. When the spectacles are removed the subjects experience similar although less marked effects.

While the basic principle of feedback applies equally to psychological and social skills the feedback can be harder to obtain and to validate. Self-awareness is a special form of feedback which helps overcome these problems.

There is general agreement that self-awareness is of value in three ways: first, it is associated with good mental health (Atkinson *et al.* 1983); second, it allows the acquisition of everyday skills (Legge and Barber, 1976), both sensory-motor and social; and third, it is a necessary step in developing the ability to form effective therapeutic and managerial relationships (Bond, 1987; Burnard 1985, 1986). This holds true for all health care workers and managers.

Awareness of Self

The term 'self-awareness' needs to be put in context as it has several possible meanings. Differentiating physical self from environment is a form of self-awareness. If I shut my dog's tail in the door, the door is not aware of this. The dog is, he knows that it is his tail and not mine. The dog's awareness may be transient and will not be of the same depth as that of a normal adult human. But nevertheless the dog has some self-awareness. At a more sophisticated level my dog does not know that it exists (as far as I can tell). While there may be no argument amongst humans that my dog exists my dog is not aware of this.

From a fairly young age a human knows both these things, that it has a body and that it exists. Within the first year of normal development an infant has begun to show signs that it has learnt that it can act on its environment and that it can control its own body. As the child grows older this knowledge becomes increasingly more sophisticated. The two basic forms of self-awareness described above (awareness of physical being and of psychological being) are an early and healthy part of development but not nearly so advanced as the kind of self-awareness which is referred to in nursing literature.

Self-awareness is more generally applied to a knowledge and understanding of the individual's own emotions, behaviour and cognition. It is however not an all-or-nothing event. Self-awareness does not suddenly occur, it needs to be developed. Even where a high degree of self-awareness has been developed it will not apply to all the components of personality and will not always be consistent over time and in differing situations.

This self-awareness occurs at a very much higher level of functioning, a level that not everyone achieves, but which can be reached with training. Figure 3.1 shows a way of structuring a hierarchy of self-awareness. This should be useful in helping to avoid confusion between different types and levels of self-awareness. Such a structure gives meaning and direction to an understanding of self-awareness.

Figure 3.1 A conceptual hierarchy of the development of self-awareness

---

Level one   Self-differentiation (a) from environment
                                    (b) from others

Level two   Self-control (a) of 'lower brain' functions
                            (b) of 'higher brain' functions

Level three Self-identification

Level four   Self-knowledge

Level five   Self-understanding

The levels identified are neither concrete nor inevitable. It may be possible to develop different levels of awareness at differing rates for various aspects of self. At different times an individual may function at higher or lower levels than usual. Adults who are well past the first stage may have difficulty in distinguishing their own feelings from those of others. Examples of this might be mass hysteria, idolizing famous people and involvement when watching films and plays and reading books. This may or may not be appropriate.

To achieve any level under particular circumstances there needs to have been acceptance of the knowledge that was gained at the previous level. This acceptance may be a matter of adjusting to the new information or may be one of changing in order to make the knowledge more acceptable. It is probable that denial interferes with the development of self-awareness and personal growth. Self-acceptance is a part of all the levels rather than a level in its own right. It is most evident at the end of level three when the person begins to accept themselves and to find a psychological place for themselves in the adult world. If acceptance at one level is incomplete then this will be reflected at higher levels. However having achieved level five at any time does not exclude functioning at a far lower level under exactly the same circumstances on another occasion.

Regression to a lower level may be voluntary, as when I take my children to the fair. To achieve the greatest fun I suspend many aspects of being a grown-up person. Regression can also be involuntary. The area which seems to cause the most problems for people is in their interpersonal relationships. Very often they have little understanding of their own behaviour or feelings until after the event, if at all. This poor performance can affect professional as well as personal relationships.

The hierarchy is described as conceptual because it is supported by no research nor any other theory. It is offered as an idea which should be criticized and hopefully developed by others.

Mental Health

Atkinson *et al.* (1983) identify self-awareness as one of six characteristics of emotional well-being. Absence of self-awareness certainly appears to be prevalent amongst those diagnosed as suffering from mental illness and those who are poorly adjusted, and seems to be an important part of many disorders. It is the aim of many therapeutic processes: analytical, cognitive and assertive training approaches, for example (Atkinson *et al.* 1983; Brown and Pedder 1975; Milne *et al.* 1985), to increase self-awareness.

It also seems true that in order to allow oneself to suffer from the more extreme effects of various abuses one would need to have rather poor self-awareness. 'Abuses' include the commonly identified abuse of alcohol, illicit drugs, solvents and smoking as well as the less commonly acknowledged but equally harmful abuses connected with diet, exercise, work, and in personal relationships. Well-developed self-awareness is a pre-requisite for having a well-adjusted personality. Someone who is well-adjusted is more able to attribute influences on their own lives to the correct cause, has better adjustment and is more able to deal with the problems of life. They will be physically and mentally healthier than others (Kabosa 1982).

There are major physical illnesses which are associated with life-style and which are preventable (Fries and Crapo 1981). Adequate self-awareness is needed to identify the need for change and to manage that change.

While the absence of self-awareness will not normally make somebody ill it is likely to be a contributing factor and will increase the chance that illness will occur and will remain.

Problem-solving

Problem-solving is a beneficial psychological skill. Instead of accepting immediate, impulsive and subjective answers to difficulties, problem-solving uses appropriate stages to arrive at a more objective position. Nurses will be familiar with problem-solving as it constitutes the framework for the theory and hopefully the practice of the nursing process.

Problem-solving can occur in a number of variations but essentially it has four stages:

(1) Assessment: identifying the need for change, the problem or the cause of the problem.
(2) Planning: deciding the likely outcomes of available action and choosing the most appropriate course of action.
(3) Implementing: carrying out the plan.
(4) Evaluation: comparing the real outcome with the intended and thus back to (1).

Self-awareness is essential in learning to solve problems. Without it objectivity can be difficult to achieve. It will also be very much more difficult to understand the need to be more objective. Some understanding and knowledge of self are essential if each of the four stages are to be effective.

In order to identify the problems or their causes the problem-solver needs to take an objective view. She will need to be aware of, acknowledge and allow for biases. This is a problem that can afflict the way doctors diagnose. There may well be a tendency for the doctor to diagnose his or her 'favourite' illness. Factors which may influence a doctor's diagnosis include such things as a belief that they are an expert in that field; preferring to look after a particular group of patients; fears and anxieties about related subjects; and unresolved conflicts related to some aspect of that illness. The tendency to be biased in diagnosis is shown by the Cleveland child abuse (Butler-Sloss 1988) affair in which two doctors diagnosed child sexual abuse at a far higher rate than had been experienced elsewhere and at other times. Many of the children diagnosed as abused were subsequently found by the courts not to have been abused and both the doctors' judgement and the technique of reflex anal dilatation were brought into doubt.

This author has never nursed a young Afro-Caribbean man who hasn't been diagnosed as schizophrenic. Of perhaps a dozen none have been diagnosed as manic-depressive, depressed, anxious or suffering from other mental illness. It is highly unlikely that all these patients were suffering from schizophrenia and would suggest that psychiatrists have a tendency to diagnose schizophrenia when symptomatology allows it, especially when treating young black males. They are for whatever reason being biased and need to increase their levels of self-awareness to become aware of it (Audley 1967). This bias may be due to differences in the way young Afro-Caribbean males experience and respond to the world when compared with the (mostly) middle-class white male doctors. It may also be caused by ignorance on the doctors' part. I know of a young Afro-Caribbean female who, following self-referral, was diagnosed as being 'pre-psychotic'.

There is nothing wrong with ignorance unless it goes unrecognized. There is work available which should help doctors (and nurses) to overcome such ignorance (Rack 1982; Shepherd and Deregowski 1981; and many articles in the *Nursing Times*).

Having successfully identified a problem, in order to decide on the most probable outcomes of actions there needs to be an accurate perception of how self (and others) will perform and respond to that action. Expectations and predictions of human behaviour must form an integral part of problem-solving simply because humans form an integral part of problems and their solutions. This applies as much to own behaviour as it does to an abstract humanity's.

In implementing a plan there needs to be feedback. People need to know how well they are getting on with the plan and how far they are from their goal. Where this is a largely technical process the feedback needs to be largely technical. When the process concerns people the feedback needs to be more about self-awareness than knowledge of results of tasks performed. However, a person performing even the most technical tasks needs to be aware of their biases. When microscopes first became good enough to allow the user to inspect human sperm it was reported that the sperm contained minute figures. The expectations of the observers had undue influence on their perception. There are enough historical examples of this for us to be certain that it is an everyday occurrence.

Evaluation too requires a good level of self-awareness for all the reasons described above. Because evaluation by its very nature implies judgement about something it is especially important that bias of any sort is avoided.

Self-awareness is especially important in learning social skills as feedback from others may be biased, open to misinterpretation, dishonest or non-existent.

Therapeutic and Managerial Relationships

A nurse has a number of resources, external and internal, available to help her care for the patients. External resources include other staff employed to support patient care and the services and materials they supply. Among the internal resources are the nurse's motivation and emotions, her knowledge of the patients and their disorders, general knowledge, especially of the social sciences, her motor, sensory and psychological skills and her experience of life.

By and large most of these resources are carefully selected and used. It is for instance not left to coincidence that a building is available and suitable to accommodate the hospital. Plans are made, experts are consulted and deliberate action taken. The outcome, however much it may be criticized, is intended. Meals are planned, cooked and served at the time of optimum benefit. However, the nurse and the hospital make less careful use of the nurse's internal resources. Very often their use seems left to chance (Hammill 1987; Hempel 1988; *Nursing Times* 1989; Priest and Woolfson 1978;

Royal Commission 1978). If a nurse happens to be sympathetic and caring all is well; if not she may be tolerated by patients and staff because she is 'efficient' or is 'like a walking text-book'. Imagine choosing a hospital building because it is 'efficient' or because it has a good library.

That social and interpersonal qualities are not always valued as they should be is a criticism of those who tolerate their absence as well as of those who lack them. Fortunately this is changing. It is increasingly recognized that human skills have therapeutic value for all patients and this principle in included in curricula and syllabi for all nurse training in the UK, and even the medical profession is beginning to look at its own practices in this area. Sadly, some of the ways that medical schools are addressing the problem are an indication of their lack of understanding. One London medical school has used actors to teach doctors interpersonal skills. This ignores one of the most important ideas behind social skills training, that social skills are not something you pretend to do, they are something the individual must develop and become more skilled at.

Use of Self

There is no concrete point at which personal skills become therapeutic, and whether professional skills are different from everyday social skills remains a matter of opinion. But it is possible that a skilled helper or therapist simply uses basic social skills in a deliberate and appropriate way more often. If this is so then becoming skilled is a matter of developing existing skills to a higher level, rather than acquiring new unknown skills. A skilled nurse uses self to achieve her aims. Use of self is about making deliberate and conscious decisions to use personal and interpersonal skills to achieve planned goals.

Unlike impulsive acts, use of self requires rational and intentional action. As skills develop their practice becomes less conscious as with most skills, although their use remains intentional.

That is not to say that interactions become manipulative. Honesty is a principle that must underlie all good nursing and managerial practice. Thought rather than reaction is implied and the skilled interactor is able to achieve a balance between spontaneity, honesty and deliberation.

Whenever opinions about others are formed they are based on previous experiences. There is a tendency to judge others by comparing others against self. The greater the difference between what is seen in others and what is seen in self the more difficult it is to understand that other person.

Forming opinions is important to all interactions. When an interactor decides that the other person is no longer attending or that he has just said the wrong thing then he is forming an opinion to that effect. What is important is to be careful of being judgemental. A statement about another person should not be a criticism, unless of course there is a specific call or compulsion to make a particular criticism. As we have seen, saying that a patient has adopted a 'sick-role' should not be an insult. It should be an observation of an event without any emotive judgement. To avoid judgement each person needs to understand self, recognizing his own prejudices and expectations. When he is able to understand how he feels an individual can be more mature about these feelings, developing or putting them into context. When this has been achieved it will be easier to accept others (i.e. to have unconditional positive regard) and to form therapeutic and managerial relationships. The care offered will not be adversely affected by own feelings.

Dexter and Wash (1986) describe psychiatric nursing by using such terms as caring, potentiating independence, restoring dignity, understanding social and psychological needs and functioning and the ability to direct skills accordingly. All these apply as much to good management as to good care and treatment. The manager will also need to share other skills with practitioners, such as problem-solving ability, assertion and high-level communication. A good degree of self-awareness is needed to develop and to practise these skills. That the principles of self-awareness should apply to managers as well as to practitioners is especially relevant as well-managed and supported staff will function more effectively and find themselves in fewer conflicts with patients, staff and the public.

DEVELOPING SELF-AWARENESS

And what of the issue of whether good nurses are born or made? I would claim that the components of myself which contribute to me being a good nurse have changed from the pre-nurse me.

Although the basic personality which was presented to the training school must have been suitable for development as a nurse I would deny that there are such things as born nurses. Good nurses require a suitable base (the personality) on which to build their skills (training). They are a product of their nature and of their environment both of which are modifiable under the right circumstances. The right circumstances include such items as adequate motivation, interest and intelligence in the learner and those items described by Fretwell (1982) and Orton (1981). They found that students felt that certain wards were of greater benefit to their learning. These wards included a democratic style of leadership, accessibility of qualified staff and openness.

The processes involved in becoming self-aware are not so simple that they can be briefly described. Burnard (1985) identifies a number of possible aspects of self-awareness. He includes elements such as thoughts, feelings, sexuality, appearance, knowledge, needs and wants, relations with others and values. Many of these occur to some extent as a normal part of life. They should also occur with greater frequency and with more intent in the professional lives of those responsible for caring for others. Such people as nurses and social workers and to some extent psychiatrists pursue an understanding of these elements as a deliberate part of their training and development.

Burnard (1985, 1986) also identifies methods associated with the development of self-awareness – group work, introspection, co-counselling, counselling, therapy, encounter/sensitivity training, self and peer assessment and evaluation and the use of video feedback.

Levels of self-awareness can be increased by using the kinds of techniques that Burnard (1985, 1986) identifies at each stage of our development (Figure 4.1) although appropriate choice will be idiosyncratic. Even the infant makes use of self-examination and introspection. What the infant has which many adults lack is the desire to explore and the ability to enjoy that exploration for its own sake. Developing self-awareness is not about leaving past levels behind. The individual should build upon the lower levels adding to his or her available resources while maintaining useful aspects and modifying those which hinder.

An individual will be better able to develop when he or she feels secure. Someone experiencing stress will tend to rely on previously learned behaviour to cope. That may not always be the most effective or constructive way to behave. Learners especially need a secure and comfortable setting with supportive peers and an experienced and competent facilitator. Confidence is essential in helping to provide that security.

A suitable ward environment has been described by Fretwell (1972) and Orton (1981). An ideal ward learning environment is created by a democratic charge nurse and includes such qualities as teamwork and effective communication. The trained nurses should be available and approachable. It seems safe to say that this is a good principle which applies to all care areas and all learners.

The greater understanding that a person has of themselves the more readily they will be able to anticipate how they will respond to different situations and thus be more able to prepare for those situations. It is also true that the greater the understanding of self the greater the understanding of others. There will therefore be greater ability to predict the behaviour, thoughts and feelings of others. While no one can be perfect it is possible for most people to improve their skills in this area as part of improving their ability to manage their own and others behaviour.

Self-assessment

One of the techniques which is essential to developing self-awareness is self-assessment and one way of practising it is through the regular use of a strengths/needs list. This can be the first stage of problem-solving.

A strengths/needs list is one way of organizing thoughts and feelings when considering change, evaluating an experience or preparing an argument. Two lists are made, one of the strengths of a situation or person, and the other of the needs of that situation or person. The strengths/needs approach specifically avoids the idea of 'weaknesses'. Apart from it being a negative and perhaps restrictive approach the weaknesses may not be relevant.

The strengths are those items which are positive, already exist and which are advantageous to the situation or person. The needs are those items which are not already present but would be counted as strengths if they were.

Strengths/needs lists can be used for evaluating situations that have been encountered and those which are expected or planned. They are a useful tool for identifying needs in an individual and as a foundation for planning change. They are best constructed by the person using them and sometimes with the help of an empathetic colleague or mentor.

By using this technique it is possible to keep a record of feelings and performance. Past and present lists can be compared to see how things have changed. Entries can be inspected with hindsight and when time has allowed objectivity. The effective use of a strengths/needs list does depend on a modicum of objectivity. One of the ways this might be checked is to compare recorded comments with what colleagues and friends say.

When learning to use a strengths/needs list it might be useful to start with a fairly simple subject. An evaluation of present working environment or a special area of interest (such as a sports team's performance). The technique of making a list can be applied to self generally or to specific areas of performance. Having identified a need the second step in problem-solving is to plan. This plan can then be implemented and evaluated.

SUMMARY

Feedback is essential to successful skills acquisition, self-awareness being especially important when learning social skills. It is also beneficial to mental health, problem-solving ability and managerial and therapeutic skills. There are five levels of self-awareness identified here. The most simple is the ability to differentiate self from the environment and other people. At its most sophisticated level it is an understanding of own emotions and how they affect behaviour. The individual can call on a number of techniques to develop self-awareness. Whichever are chosen the individual needs to feel supported and secure in order to develop. A useful basic tool is the strengths/needs list.

4 Interactions

TRANSACTIONAL ANALYSIS

It is during interactions with others that most difficult behaviour arises. Fortunately this is when a skilled interactor is able to assert the most influence.

One of the more successful theories of interaction is Transactional Analysis (commonly known as TA). TA is described in the book *Games People Play* (Berne 1966). It is essentially a Freudian/psychoanalytical theory.

While a useful way of looking at transactions it has three main drawbacks which limit its use: first, it is too complex to be easily and widely understood and used; second, it can, because of its Freudian heritage, present a rather pessimistic view of humanity; and third, it is subjective as it relies heavily on the interpretation of the practitioner.

The problem of its complexity can be overcome by using only the basic positions described by Berne (1966). A more positive view can be encouraged by describing interactions rather than transactions and it can be most usefully applied as a means of self-evaluation. When used in this way it might be described as 'interactional evaluation'. While this presents a very simple model it serves as a useful introduction to the study of interactions.

The Positions

Figure 4.1 shows the three positions of parent, adult and child diagrammatically represented as three circles while Figure 4.2 shows some of the negative and positive qualities of the parent, the adult and the child. These qualities are a normal and healthy part of everyone's personality.

Figure 4.1   Diagrammatic representation of the parent, the adult and the child

---

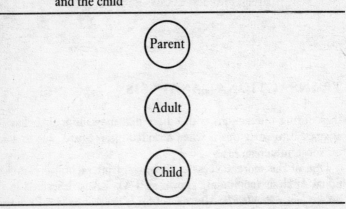

The Child   The greater portion of responses and reactions to the world are acquired in childhood. It is a period in which the child acquires, practises and develops the ways in which he or she deals with the world and with self into adult life.

The ways that a person deals with the world might be described as strategies. An example of the child's strategy is that when confronted with a critical ward sister, Student Nurse Clare tends to become sullen and silent. This is the way she deals with criticism. An alternative strategy might be to become defensive and then critical of others in order to defend against criticism. These strategies are learned in early childhood. Student Nurse Clare probably learnt that the best way to deal with her parents' criticism was to keep quiet and sulk. This is an example of the negative 'child'. It is that part of personality that sulks and has tantrums, it is demanding and wants all its needs and desires fulfilled.

There is also a positive side to the child. It is that part of the person which enjoys playing. It has lots of fun, takes risks and likes to explore and experiment for the fun of it. The positive child puts on funny hats at the ward party and does things like playing minor jokes on colleagues and staff which might at times be on the edge of social acceptability. In many cultures, including those dominant in

Figure 4.2 Some of the negative and positive qualities of the parent, the child and the adult

	Positive	Negative
Parent	caring comforting reassuring takes responsibility encouraging	patronizing directive bossy intolerant authoritarian judgemental
Child	playful adventurous humorous exploring trusting	demanding selfish sulky greedy teasing
Adult	reasonable subjective responsible for self assertive a decision-maker respectful empathetic genuine tactful	Inappropriate when used on such occasions as a party or when giving care to someone in need of positive parenting

Europe and the English-speaking parts of the world, it is the child in us which is the most neglected part of the individual. The positive child is an important part of the nurse's repertoire (Niven 1989).

The Parent As an individual grows he or she begins to acquire aspects of parenthood. At an early stage he or she observes this in parents and practises it in games. These games eventually become reality. Even if the grown person does not become a parent there will be many parts of his or her behaviour which are similar in appearance and function to a parent's.

The negative parent is patronizing. It is that part of the person that assumes it knows better and makes ready judgements of others and of self. Feelings of guilt are associated with the parent.

The positive parent is that part which cares for others. When the child is in need of care it is the parent which reassures and makes things all right. It is the positive parent that constructs boundaries and limits behaviour.

Nurses for obvious reasons find themselves in the position of parent on many occasions and have a duty to ensure that they interact from the position of the positive parent.

The Adult The adult is the objective, reasonable and realistic part of personality. The most important function of the adult is to use its objectivity to decide which approach is most appropriate. The adult recognizes there are times when it must give way to the child – at a party, for example – and to the parent – when telling a child off. It is also responsible for asserting itself at the appropriate time, something which is difficult for the child and the parent to do. There is no negative or positive adult. It is instead either appropriate or inappropriate. The adult position is the most appropriate to adopt when dealing with the difficult patient.

There are times when the negative child or the negative parent are appropriate, and it should not be forgotten that both the negative and the positive aspects are part of normal and healthy development. It is also normal to be inappropriate in the position adopted. One of the skills that a nurse should possess is that she is more able to adopt the most useful position.

THE NURSE'S INTERACTIONS

An interaction between two people can be represented as shown in Figure 4.3.

The interactions between the two are represented by the lines passing from the left to the right. Those lines which pass through the centre of the diagram mark successful interaction. The positions of the two people are complementary and they are likely to achieve something as a result of their interaction. These lines are

Figure 4.3   An interaction between two people

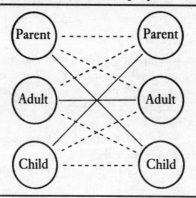

shown as solid. The interactions are balanced.

Those interactions which are not likely to be successful are represented by the broken lines, which do not pass through the centre. These interactions are unbalanced. The positions that the two people adopt are not complementary. Of course there will be times when these 'unbalanced' interactions are successful – at a party or during a game the interactions will be much more fun if they are child–child.

When the nurse adopts the parent position she increases the possibility that the patient will respond by adopting the child position. This will be useful when it is appropriate for the nurse to be the positive parent and the patient the positive child, but many patients will be unwilling or unable to adopt the positive child position. They will instead be negative or parental.

Most people will find the negative parent provocative. Likewise, should the nurse approach the situation from the position of the child it becomes likely that the patient will become parental. Even where the nurse and the patient are in complementary positions they may be acting inappropriately. All this increases the chance that the interaction will become difficult. The more intractable the difficulties become the more likely it is that aggression and violence will occur. The nurse who is patronizing or demanding is making a major contribution to the negative behaviour of the 'difficult' patient.

The Nurse's Position

A charge nurse working on a medical ward has many roles to fulfil. Some of the patients feel very insecure. They are unsure of what is happening to them and need someone to accept some of the responsibility for their care. To them she is the 'parent', they are in the child position. She fulfils some of the roles or functions that their parents fulfilled for them when they were children. She reassures them, makes sure they are comfortable, warm and fed and attends to their illness, pain and care. On this occasion, the relationship is positive and by and large appropriate. By providing a secure environment the charge nurse is making it easier for the patients to develop their independence and move from a child to an adult position. However if a patient does not conform to the expectations of the ward staff, refuses to take a particular medicine, for example, and the charge nurse adopts an 'I know better than you and you had better do as you are told or else' approach, standing over the patient with hands on hips and frowning, she is then being patronizing. This is the negative parent.

Adopting the parent position will only be successful if the patient is in the child position.

The charge nurse also has to deal with senior staff of all professions. If the senior nurse is particularly authoritarian then she may well be in the parent position when dealing with her juniors. If the charge nurse adopts a child position – allowing or even expecting someone to tell her what to do, then this interaction will be successful. Doctors are very much in the parent position. In order for the medical system in hospitals to work all participants must behave as if the doctors are the parents. They know best, are the only people who are able to make important decisions about other people (often with little or no cooperation from others) and will not be told anything. Doctors very much adopt the parent position when interacting with nurses. The following example illustrates the parent position. Many nurses have confirmed that they have experienced a similar situation.

Dr X arrives on the ward just as lunches have been served and announces to a staff nurse that he will see Mrs Smith. Mrs Smith has not eaten properly for several days and is now attempting her first meal. This is explained to Dr X who says that he is busy and he will have to see her now and that staff nurse should go and get her. The doctor is adopting a very negative parent position. The staff nurse has three positions available to her. She can use the child position and respond by doing as she is told with either good or bad grace, and she might have a tantrum complaining that the doctor is making things hard for her. She could adopt the parent position and tell the doctor that this really is not good enough and that he is being most unreasonable and cannot see Mrs Smith. Her third option is to be adult. As an adult she will tell the doctor in a calm manner that Mrs Smith is attempting her first meal for several days and that it is important she be allowed to continue. Additionally, if Dr X can make time available later, she will have Mrs Smith ready and waiting for him.

The child position is the complementary one in this case. If the nurse adopts this position the interaction will be successful – the doctor and nurse will have communicated in such a way and taken such action as to carry through the interaction to a conclusion. The nurse may not like it but will have acted in a way that conformed to the doctor's wish. The doctor may even feel pleased that the nurse is obedient.

Adopting the child position however may have long-term consequences which are unacceptable to the nurse and to the doctor. First, the nurse may be adding to her own stress by carrying out instructions she does not approve of. While disagreeing with the doctor may also be stressful it will, over a long period, be less harmful. Lack of control over own actions is associated with higher stress levels (Geer and Maisel, 1972; Kabosa, Kahn and Maddi, 1982; Seligman, 1975; Seligman *et al.*, 1975) and in this case the situation remains unresolved. Second, the unsatisfactory situation of a doctor interfering with a patient's well-being is perpetuated and in this respect the nurse may well be acting in an unprofessional manner. The doctors may want an obedient nurse when they are present and want something, but presumably when they have gone home or to other wards they want the ward to be staffed by competent, mature and responsible nurses. This contradiction between demanding obedience on the one hand and competence and initiative on the other is one of the difficulties of adopting the parent position.

This contradiction is evident in real parent–child relationships. Parents tend to make demands on children which contradict their expectations of those children. When a mother or father tells a teenager that they should be more mature and act their age they are often contradicting themselves. Mature people do not have to do as their parents tell them and a child who is acting their age will certainly not be mature. It might be more appropriate to tell the teenager that they are still a child and must behave accordingly.

If the nurse adopts a parent position she will tell the doctor that he cannot possibly see Mrs Smith for the reasons described above and that anyway he should know better. He had better come back later. This interaction will not be successful. Unless one person or the other climbs down the relationship will be almost unsalvageable and there will be repercussions on those involved. Unfortunately most senior staff have committed themselves to a system which reinforces the doctor's position and it is easier and safer to treat the nurse as the wrongdoer and the doctor as faultless.

The most appropriate action is for the nurse to be adult. In doing this she will effectively communicate with the doctor in an unprovocative way while maintaining her professionalism. She is acting in both her own and the patient's best interests. If the doctor then chooses to react badly it is his responsibility, but he will have fewer grounds for complaint and is more likely to modify his behaviour in the future. By being adult the nurse will allow the doctor a way out of the conflict.

An ideal situation would be for all professional interactions to be adult to adult. These interactions would be mature, objective and reasonable. It is however unrealistic to expect everyone to be adult all the time. Humans have many emotions, most of which are 'good', although some are 'bad'. It is difficult to have any great degree of control over emotions. The nurse has to strive to be as adult as is possible without losing her humanity. To some extent, this is what being professional is about.

There will also be times when it is not in the patient's interests for the nurse to be adult. Where a patient has been involved in a road traffic accident and is suffering from several injuries he is confused, in pain and unsure of himself. He does not know what to expect or what is expected of him. Any ideas he does have may be inaccurate. He needs pain relief, reassurance and to be helped to understand what is happening. It is in order, and indeed necessary, for the nurse to be parental. But the negative patronizing parent will cause great difficulties for the patient. He will have less understanding of what is happening and will suffer from his contact with the nurse rather than benefit from it.

Some weeks later the patient is recovering, getting ready to go home. He is now a more active and assertive individual who understands his experience and has a large degree of control over himself and his life. He is far more able to fulfil his own needs. It would now be quite wrong for the nurse to adopt a parental approach to this man. He should be treated like an adult. There should be no assumption on the nurse's part that she knows better than he what is good for him, or that the decisions he has to make about his own life are right or wrong. By treating the patient as an adult the nurse will be more able to give him appropriate advice about his after-care and future. If he is treated in an adult manner he will respond in a much more positive way.

The change from a parent–child relationship to an adult–adult relationship will not normally be sudden but appear as the relationship develops. Any child or parent components in their relationship should be positive and the trend should be towards as much adultness as is useful as soon as is possible.

Adultness as a Tool

We are not in any one position at a time. Our interactions will be mixtures of parent, adult and child positions. We might approach an interaction from a predominantly adult position but there will be elements of parent and child in it. We can, for example, while having a very adult-adult interaction with a patient, have a joke with him and also show concern for his welfare.

This modification of TA gives a simple tool to help develop an overall approach to interactions. As the interactions become more and more skilled and sophisticated, it becomes harder and harder to fit them into any simple theory. An alternative way to describe 'adultness' is as 'assertiveness' (Bond 1987). Those wishing to develop their interpersonal, therapeutic and aggression management skills to a higher level are well advised to pursue assertion through a formal training course as well as doing further reading and practice.

SUMMARY

Berne's Transactional Analysis can be modified to give a more easily used method of evaluating own interactions. Interactions can be described in terms of the positions that can be adopted. These are the parent, the child and the adult positions. The nurse should strive to have adult-adult interactions with her colleagues and patients although at times it may be appropriate to be a caring parent or a playful child. Adopting the adult position will improve all nursing and reduce the possibility of the nurse provoking difficult behaviour in others. This will also help her to manage difficulties when they arise.

5 Difficult Behaviour

SUBJECTIVITY

The labelling of behaviour as difficult is subjective and depends on the personalities, roles and social skills of the interacters. Behaviour which one person finds intolerable may be seen as desirable by another. Likewise behaviour which is difficult under some circumstances may be acceptable under others.

The following exercise is aimed at helping people to recognize that even the most difficult person is not very different from everybody else.

A group of learners are first asked to make a list of the qualities they find difficult in other people. It is essential that all the participants understand what they list is not to be regarded as either right or wrong. When this list has been prepared it is transferred to a board, duplications are erased and any queries clarified.

The learners are then asked to go through the list and count how many of the items apply to themselves at some time or another. It is usual for most people to 'own' all but a few of the items. Typically out of about thirty items the range of ownership is from twenty-two to twenty-eight. There are invariably some items which cannot be admitted. Females cannot admit to being male chauvinists and people who never drink cannot own to 'drunkenness'.

It becomes quite clear that many of the qualities that are difficult in others can be found in everybody. However, many patients who are very difficult are quantitatively different from most other people. The majority of people become drunk to some degree at some point in life, but their behaviour remains markedly different from that of a chronic alcoholic and as a rule they do not become violent. Likewise, although having the potential, most people do not normally without provocation become abusive, violent, sullen, manipulative, etc.

There are some people who are difficult because of their personality and others who are difficult because of the circumstances in which they find themselves. There may be little difference in how they are being difficult and in how much self-control they have. If a nurse can understand that a man is abusive because he has become angry as a result of recent experience she is more able to react in the most suitable way. If she is aware that his abusiveness is a result of his negative attitude towards other people, his lack of respect for others and his almost overwhelming need to have his own way, then she may take a completely different approach.

There are a number of ways at looking at what it is that makes someone difficult. Most obviously it is easy to say that the individual is a difficult person (if we are polite). It may also be that it is a failure to tolerate them that is the problem. These two views may at times be accurate. When someone is being difficult it is most likely that they are displaying behaviour which is far from ideal and that others find this particular behaviour especially difficult.

Each person is responsible for their own behaviour. I personally find over-dramatic people almost intolerable whatever they are doing. Not only do they have a problem with the way they present themselves but I have a problem with the way I feel about the way they present themselves. This problem may be mutual and left alone can lead to an irresolvable conflict.

It is usually to my advantage and in the interest of society to have as little conflict as possible. If I am in conflict with my neighbour I have no special responsibility to resolve the conflict, although for my own benefit I should seek to resolve my conflicts with other members of the public, but when I am acting as a nurse I do have a special responsibility (UKCC 1984).

In an interaction with a patient I have to accept that I am the professional and the person who is best equipped to take a lead. In addition, as a nurse I am being paid to provide a service to the patient and have a responsibility to promote successful interactions with each patient I meet.

When having an interaction with a patient the nurse also has a vested interest in a positive outcome. The more positive she is about the relationship and the more successful she is the more rewarding she will find her interactions. Difficult people are often so because they are discontented, frustrated and defensive. Being difficult often leads to feelings of discontentment, frustration and vulnerability.

There may be occasions when it is necessary to be difficult. As a charge nurse I resisted those things in the institution which I saw as being against the best interests of the patients and staff within my area of responsibility. As the nurse in charge I had responsibility for the well-being of everybody on the ward. On many occasions in fulfilling that responsibility I am sure I was seen as difficult by my seniors. This was as much because I had raised an issue as for the way the senior nurse felt about the issue. When a nurse finds herself in conflict with her seniors or with other non-nursing colleagues it is important that she avoids unnecessary conflict. If she can confront her senior nurse, for example, without adding personal conflict to the professional conflict then she has a far greater chance of success.

It is wrong for nurses to avoid being difficult at all costs. There are times when they have a duty to confront and complain, but in a professional manner. Managers and administrators find the quiet compliant nurse who ignores problems less difficult than the active assertive nurse who identifies and highlights problems. But it is part of the nurse's role to question and to present their own professional opinion.

If we accept that some nurse-created difficulties are justified then we must allow that the same applies to the patient. Indeed many patients feel threatened by their situation and may well behave in a manner which they believe increases the chance of prompt and effective treatment. This sort of behaviour may well be difficult for the nurse. Where that behaviour arises from an evident cause it is easier to tolerate. Where a parent has brought an injured child into A&E it is understandable that they may become very demanding and intolerant of delay. Where an apparently healthy young man makes great demands and behaves as if his cut finger was a major disaster tolerance is more difficult. Do the two (parent and young man) feel any different from each other? Experience of being a patient and of being a nurse suggests to me that the majority of complaints the patients make against the service and those who are a part of it are justified. Even those that may not be justified from an objective viewpoint are often justifiable from the patient's point of view.

When groups of learners are asked to list the things in others that they find difficult they come up with a great variety of items ranging from the very specific ('people who push') to the very general ('men' or 'mothers'). These choices cannot be disputed. An expression of what a person finds difficult has to be accepted as true, even if some of the items may seem strange to others.

Identifying the reasons why behaviour is seen as difficult is another question. Why does it matter if a person pushes another, why is it difficult to interact with someone who is shouting or with someone who will not shout. One person might find another difficult because they are threatening, competitive or stressful.

Threatening Behaviour

The behaviour of another person might sometimes appear to present a threat. This threat may be actual or anticipated, it may be acute or chronic, it may be against our physical or our mental well-being and it may be a threat to do something or not to do something. What will be important is that there is a perception of a threat rather than a definite threat.

A threat by a healthy young man to do damage is an actual threat. It is acute and is primarily against physical well-being. A change in working conditions forced by a manager is usually an anticipated chronic threat against mental well-being. Very often a threat can be implied, anticipated or imagined. It is then just as real to the victim as an actual threat. Talk of someone being 'insecure' or 'resistant to change' is an identification of it. Although the threat is not actual the person is reacting as if it is.

If an individual's mother or father has been particularly authoritarian then that person may experience the threat as feelings of suppression or rejection when interacting with people who remind them of that parent. When someone is described as difficult they are being attributed with threatening behaviour, but if there was no threat involved their behaviour would be no problem. It may be that they are responding to a threat that they perceive in the behaviour of other people. A nurse may often participate in activities which make her patients feel threatened. Some nurses also behave in an overtly threatening manner.

Competitive Behaviour

Another way to view experience of difficult people is to consider the conflicting needs that arise for different people in an interaction.

A nurse will have her own needs. She will need to achieve or avoid certain things to feel satisfied. The need to lead a life free of unnecessary work is evident in many people including some nurses. This may well produce a tendency in the nurse to under-react to patients' needs. A simple task in any out-patients' or A&E department is to notify the patients of the waiting time. In many departments this is too much effort and patients who make such demands are seen as unreasonable. Where needs coincide interactions are easy, but where there is a conflict of needs the individuals involved may feel a need to compete in order to fulfil their own need. A patient may feel that the only way to achieve the care he thinks he needs is to be competitive. He may feel that other patients are depriving him of attention or may try to put himself in a superior position to the nurse in the hierarchy. The greater the conflict the greater the difficulty in interacting.

Stressful Behaviour

Another way to think about interactions is to view as difficult any interaction which causes the nurse to feel stressed. The most probable cause of stress is threat to well-being. It might however be more acceptable for a nurse to describe herself or another as being stressed than to talk of a threat. For instance, someone who talks non-stop and at great length is only threatening in that they are interfering with other work. To confront them in any way might lead to unpleasantness and bring ridicule on those associated with them. Anyone who behaves like this is seen as being different and a problem. Again, having a 'conversation' with someone who rushes on regardless is stressful because there will be a conflict between the patient's need to talk and the nurse's need to do other work, have their own say and avoid extra problems.

Except in special circumstances it is invariably true that nurses have to exercise a degree of administrative responsibility. This may often include restricting the behaviour of others by, for example, enforcing a non-smoking policy or not allowing patients to wander willy-nilly from ward to ward. While the nurse no doubt regards the patients who behave like this as difficult it may well be that the patient sees the nurse or those the nurse represents as being difficult because they attempt to restrict him or her.

The way the individual experiences difficulty will vary as will the way he or she individually describes that experience. A nurse describing a patient as difficult may be talking about the same thing as a nurse who describes a patient as being stressful, demanding, and so on.

It would be useful if there was a common understanding of the things that people do when they are being difficult, and a good start is the assumption that it is not what they do but the way they do it which is important. It is the way that people present themselves and their message which make them threatening, competitive or stressful to interact with. For instance, if I am stopped by a traffic policeman and treated with some respect (as an adult) I feel more able to treat him with respect and so our interaction is more likely to be successful. I will be more influenced by his message and he will be less likely to report me. If on the other hand the police officer is patronizing or rude I will react in a less favourable manner and our interaction will be less successful. I will be less influenced by his message and he is more likely to report me. It is not what the police officer does but the way he does it that is important.

WAYS OF BEING DIFFICULT

Most difficult behaviour will fall into one or more of five categories: withdrawal, passivity, manipulation, aggression and violence. These can be defined:

(a) Withdrawal is the act of refusing to interact.
(b) Passivity is the failure to take any action.
(c) Manipulation is the practice of using devious and dishonest means.
(e) Aggression is the expression of anger with an implication of violence.
(f) Violence is a physical act against others, self or property which is intended to or causes damage.

As a general rule interactions are difficult because of the qualities of both people involved although this may not always be true. Where a nurse has approached an interaction in an adult manner and has avoided any of the ways of being difficult, she has been reasonable. However some individuals are unable to respond in an adult manner whatever the approach so that having fulfilled her responsibility to be as adult as possible the nurse may still find that the other person responds in a difficult way. A good example of this is when a nurse points something out to a doctor in an adult manner and the doctor responds badly. I have worked with more than one consultant of whom it was said if you wanted him to do something you should ask for the opposite. The consultants in question appeared to hold the view that they were the boss and that only they had the skills and knowledge to make decisions. Any demonstration of ability by nurses was seen as a threat and treated as such. Some nurses also feel and behave like this.

Withdrawal

This is the act of refusing to interact. There are some circumstances in which it is normal not to interact with the other people present. Anyone who travels on public transport is by and large expected to keep to themselves. Patients sitting in queues in an out-patients department generally do not interact. There may be transitory interactions when people have to pass each other or if something unusual happens but for most of the time no interaction takes place. It would become a problem if this behaviour was continued when people were approached by the staff and in the consulting rooms.

Not all withdrawal behaviour is so gross or so automatic. Very often the withdrawal may be partial. As a student nurse in the early 1970s it was made quite clear to me that on no occasion should I hold the hand of, or put my arms around, a female patient. The fear was that the action could be misinterpreted by an observer! Like most of my colleagues I soon overcame this training and was able to comfort those who needed it by touching and holding them without feeling threatened. The nurses had been taught to withdraw from physical contact with the patient. Withdrawn behaviour is often self-inflicted and is a way of distancing self from feelings in others which cause one discomfort. It is in the same class as the common reaction of telling someone, 'There, there, don't cry.'

There are times when a person may refuse to interact for moral reasons. Refusing to talk to someone who has reported another nurse or refusing to have anything to do with a nurse who is manipulative are both acts of withdrawal. One of the problems with withdrawing for moral reasons is that these are generally very subjective and fail to take account of all the factors affecting the others involved. Withdrawal for moral reasons will tend to polarize people towards one extreme of opinion or the other.

Passivity

This is the failure to take any action and is different from withdrawal in that a passive person is often willing to allow interactions to take place and indeed relies upon others involved in the interaction as a means of remaining passive. This may on occasion be deliberate but the result is that others find themselves making decisions and taking action for the passive person. Institutionalization is a form of chronic passivity. A person suffering from institutional neurosis allows all decisions to be made and all basic (usually physical) needs to be met by the institution. This process is circular in that a passive person allows it to happen and institutionalization leads to passivity. This is often what is mistakenly meant by 'the sick role'. The patient becomes dependent on the everyday skills of others and is increasingly unable to fulfil their needs by their own actions. Many of the simple physical tasks remain unaffected but higher functions like decision-making are lost altogether.

This category has many degrees. Many patients are passive only in certain respects, for instance, in the view that nurses and doctors know best. Again, there may be occasions when passivity is a deliberate choice. A nurse is a member of a team and may find that she disagrees with the decisions of the team. On such occasions she may feel that it is best to go along with everybody else without expressing her own view. She is being passive, but if she makes a deliberate decision to keep her views to herself she is being less passive.

There may be occasions when it is best to be passsive, as in a medical emergency when the staff may be more able to go about their business if the patient has a degree of passivity. On a busy ward, staffed by old-fashioned nurses passivity is often considered a desirable quality and a degree of passivity is essential in those lower down the hierarchy of the medical model of care. However being passive has little long-term therapeutic value. The aim of all good health and social care must be to develop in the patient/client an optimum degree of independence. Independence and passivity are not compatible.

It is very sad to see patients becoming passive but even more so when it happens to a nurse. Nursing is about being active and one of the worst things to afflict a team of nurses is apathy. This may be the result of stress-related burn-out, poor management or failure of the team process. Passivity is one of the greatest forms of neglect in nursing and gives rise to all kinds of difficult behaviour in colleagues and patients.

Manipulation

This is the practice of using devious and dishonest means. The most obvious example of it is 'attention seeking' behaviour. 'Attention seeking' implies that the individual needs attention from others and will commit various acts (sometimes dishonest) to force others to fulfil that need. In its most cynical form it assumes that the attention of the staff is important in its own right and that possessing that attention has a value. Standard nursing response used to be to ignore the patient as much as possible in the hope that he or she would learn that 'attention seeking' was a waste of time. The more enlightened view is that some patients need reassurance because of specific events in their life or because of the way they feel about life in general. In order to get this reassurance the individual uses (often unconsciously) things like minor physical ailments as a means of getting others to tell them everything will be all right. Modern nursing approach must be able to offer unconditional and appropriate reassurance so that the reassurance seeking patient is able to understand that there is little need to behave in this way.

Sometimes patients are more direct in their searching and will make overt demands on the staff. Whether or not the staff like this, it is far more constructive. A patient who is unable to function without staff support is being passive. It is only when they begin to disguise their passivity that it can be said that they are being manipulative.

Manipulation is a poor substitute for honesty. It is a way of avoiding the danger of confrontation or of gaining something without due effort. A very good example of a manipulative approach was that of the RCN during the 1988 ballot on industrial action. When members were asked to vote on whether industrial action was to be allowed, a statement concerning danger to patients was included. The only way to express a belief that industrial action should be an option was to express a wish to endanger patients. Surprisingly most members went along with this approach. Nurses are wrong not to object to anything but positive and open management and leadership. They are even more in the wrong if they adopt a manipulative approach towards their patients.

The main problem with manipulative behaviour is that it is stressful and can distract the attention of the nurses from the patient's real problem. Doctors and nurses will be familiar with patients who undergo repeated physical examination for some bodily complaint in spite of there being no evidence that anything is wrong. The patient appears to be unable to express their psychological needs directly. Likewise a manipulative nurse may distract managers, colleagues and patients from their real tasks.

Positive use of manipulation includes placebos, some experimental techniques and helping staff to overcome resistance to change by deliberately managing the rate of change. What makes this form of manipulation acceptable to most people is that the manipulator must come clean after the event. For instance only rarely and with third party approval should patients never be told that they were on a placebo. Indeed most of the benefit of using a placebo is to enable the patient to be confronted with the fact.

Aggression

There is a lot of nonsense talked about aggression, which is the expression of anger with an implication of violence. On the one hand there is a body of opinion which holds that aggression is an inevitable part of human life arising from an aggressive drive, and on the other there are those who express the idea that humanity can overcome all its aggression and live in eternal peaceful coexistence. Others express the belief that humans are the most aggressive animal on earth or that violence on television 'makes' people violent.

Quite clearly humanity does have some innate capacity for aggression (along with every other form of animal life and some plants). Equally clearly there is an element of environmental effect and individuals do reflect the level of aggression they have encountered in life. Everyone has the ability to be aggressive under the right circumstances. Unfortunately some individuals have an abnormally aggressive range of responses. The causes may be biological – abnormal variation and brain damage, for example. While brain damage does not necessarily cause a change in personality it might lead to loss of self-control, less inhibitions and greater frustration.

There are some individuals who have been so damaged by their experience of life that they are overly aggressive in most of their interactions and are easily provoked. This might be because they have learnt as a child that aggression pays off or it might be because they have unacknowledged feelings about the things they have experienced. These feelings remain and build up until a trigger sets off an aggressive reaction. For instance, often adult child-abusers have been abused as children (Kemp and Kemp 1978). It may be that the experience of being the object of aggression increases the possibility of being aggressive. Additionally aggressive adults can act as a model for a child's behaviour (Asch 1952).

The way an individual expresses aggressive feelings varies with personality. Not all expressions of anger, rage and so on will be loud or active. Sometimes they may be expressed by sullenness or dumb rage.

It must be remembered that there are times when aggression is of vital importance. In defending self, family and property against attack there are times when an aggressive individual will fare better than a passive one. At times of natural or man-made disaster an aggressive determination might increase the chance of survival. Where humans still have to catch their food aggression will give them an edge over their prey and competitors. Being adult and being civilized is about learning to control aggression and to use it appropriately. It is those who have little or no control over their aggression who are the most difficult.

Violence

Violence is different to aggression and is a physical act against others, self or property which is intended to or causes damage. Aggression is a feeling or a drive which leads to the individual being in a state in which they are more prepared to act. Violence is one of the ways in which the individual may then act (the others being fleeing and freezing). Violence has essentially two forms which are given various names. They are perhaps most usefully identified as instrumental and expressive. Instrumental violence is that used to achieve something. A soldier uses instrumental violence as does someone defending themselves from attack, a sportsman putting that extra something into avoiding defeat and a businessman getting the best deal.

Expressive violence is the ventilation of feelings without regard to their effect. Vandalism, domestic violence and self-harm are examples.

Sometimes violence may be both instrumental and expressive. Smacking a naughty child contains both instrumental and expressive elements. To be entirely instrumental (cold-blooded) or entirely expressive (without any intention) is a waste of time.

In its more acceptable form violence arises out of a need to achieve a specific goal. Such violence might be associated with defence or with taking possession of something. If anyone doubts that this is a more acceptable form of violence consider the expressions 'mindless' and 'gratuitous' violence. Where violence is committed without great gain it is socially less acceptable. Robbing an old lady of fifty pence is seen as worse than robbing an old lady of £50,000, even though (and perhaps especially when) the violence involved in the robbery is the same. Society, of which everyone is a part, seems to be more ready to forgive violent crime that might have been worth it. Football hooligans get far worse press than armed robbers.

Acts of 'mindless' violence are usually an expression of a general feeling of dissatisfaction, alienation or frustration. This is often expressed through non-gaining crime – vandalism, hooliganism and the theft of small items by people well able to afford to pay for them. Violence which is presumably 'mindful' is aimed at some gain – robbery, resisting arrest or protection.

This also applies to violent acts against the person. It seems that to rape an attractive young woman is less of a crime than to rape an unattractive elderly woman. This may be because there is more sympathy in our legal and journalistic systems for someone who is overcome by lust at the sight of a desirable woman. That same system cannot understand how anyone can be so depraved as to rape an old woman who is not sexually attractive (and is presumably not a sex object). A more humane view might be that robbing an old lady of her last penny is the same whether that be a part of fifty pence of fifty pounds. She still has nothing left. On the other hand can it be said that a robber who takes only half the money available is only half as much a criminal? What is relevant is not the act of violence (and rape is an act of violence not of lust) but its effects on the victim. Striking me on the chin during a mugging is less of a crime than striking an old lady or a child in the same situation.

Being male I have a heavier chin than most females and being a young adult I am in better health and less fragile than the old lady.

The child may be less fragile than me but I am far more able to adjust to the assault than a child.

Additionally males have more experience at dealing with violence because it is an important part of being a schoolboy (Archer and Westerman 1981). The rough and tumble of the playground or sports field helps the growing boy to develop a balanced view of aggression and violence. He can more easily understand that aggression can be enjoyable or painful depending on how it is used. This makes violence less threatening for most men. Most difficulties arise from bullying which is not the same as rough and tumble. It is often adult bullies who present problems for others. Having a bit of a wrestle with someone at a party after a row is not the same kind of violence as bullying. Bullying is about using violence in order to have a detrimental effect on others. It can be used in both expressive and in instrumental violence.

As with aggression an important element of violence is loss of control. Most violence encountered at work by nurses is as a result of the assailant losing self-control. The assailant does not set out to commit a violent act and however inevitable it may be it is probable that the assailant does not wish to be violent. They cannot help themselves and are quite clearly in a different category to most other violent criminals who are able to meditate upon and to anticipate their crime.

This loss of control, while at times being quite horrific, is to the nurse's advantage. There is little that a nurse can do to prevent someone from committing a determined and premeditated act of violence. However a skilled nurse can have a great influence over someone who is struggling to maintain their control. Nurses can best protect themselves (and others) by helping a violent person to keep or regain control. This applies equally to people who cause damage to themselves and who damage property (perhaps in an attempt to avoid harm to others).

SUMMARY

The labelling of someone as being difficult arises from the individual's perception of the situation. Personality and role play a major part in shaping those perceptions. Everybody can be difficult at times. Nurses are no exception to this. It is very often a feeling of threat which makes behaviour seem difficult.

There are a number of ways in which behaviour is difficult. These are identified here as withdrawal, passivity, manipulation, aggression and violence.

6 Managing Difficult Behaviour

WITHDRAWAL

Withdrawal is the act of refusing to interact. It is best managed by building a relationship with the patient. This relationship will be more difficult to achieve where the nurse has for example to force life-saving measures upon the patient. Generally the patient will respond positively to being treated with respect, empathy and genuineness. This includes understanding the patient's need for 'space' and allowing them privacy. Even when the patient is unwilling to respond they should still be offered an explanation of what is happening and what will happen to them. If cared for by a nurse using a positive parent and an adult approach the withdrawn patient will slowly begin to develop trust in the nurse and be able to risk interacting. It is essential to remember that a withdrawn patient will still be alert and that their observation and memory skills will still be intact. It is important to consider physical and neurological examination when deciding on the cause of the withdrawal. It may be a result of physical disorder, shock, an impending or recent fit or an overdose of drugs.

PASSIVITY

Passivity is a failure to take any action and can be a symptom of depression, of institutionalization and of 'burn-out'. Again the cornerstones of a caring approach are most appropriate – respect, empathy and genuineness. The passive individual needs to be encouraged to try out new ways of behaving without feeling under undue pressure. They too need careful physical investigation to exclude physical factors before they are treated as being in a primarily psychological state. Someone who is being passive might be suffering from anaemia or similar nutritional deficiency either as a cause or a result of their passivity. Similarly some medication especially those used in psychiatry can produce a decline in motivation.

MANIPULATION

Manipulation, the practice of using devious and dishonest means, is much more provocative than withdrawal and passivity. It often appears to be more deliberate and controlled. The patient may however have very little control over this kind of behaviour. It might have been their strategy for surviving a difficult life and is therefore an habitual and perhaps safe way to behave. It is essential that the nurse uses three qualities when managing manipulation. She must be genuine – not allowing herself to become involved in 'games'. She must also make sure that she retains a good degree of objectivity, not allowing her frustration to distance her from the patient. It is also important that good communications are maintained amongst the care team in order to minimize the adverse effects of the manipulation.

AGGRESSION AND VIOLENCE

Aggression is the expression of anger with an implication of violence. Violence is a physical act against others, self or property which is intended to cause damage. Both aggression and violence are a special case as they present very similar problems. They are more threatening than passivity, withdrawal and manipulation. Aggression and violence are often used as interchangeable terms but they are quite different phenomena. Aggression is a feeling which often shows itself in behaviour while violence is an act. They can occur together but aggression more often occurs without violence. The effects on the victim can be similar. While the physical results of violence are usually visible the psychological effects can go unrecognized. Aggressive behaviour, such as threats or uncontrolled expression of anger, can also have far-reaching results. It is vital that nurses learn to prevent aggressive and violent behaviour whoever the perpetrator or the victim. When confronted with aggression and violence the nurse can cope with it, deal with it or manage it.

PREVENTING DIFFICULT BEHAVIOUR

Prevention is the best approach to life's difficulties. Fire prevention saves more lives than fire-fighting. This also applies to violence and aggression. It ought to be true of health care in general but is not, as far as official organizations in this country are concerned. This is significant because a healthier population ought to be a less aggressive one. While effective action should prevent nearly all impending aggression it must be remembered that the aggression which still occurs becomes disproportionately dangerous if it is unexpected and staff are unprepared for it.

Some forms of prevention, when used in isolation, aggravate the situation. Deterrence is usually a waste of time. If guards were introduced in A&E departments as the only method of preventing violence some individuals would direct their aggression elsewhere and some might arm themselves in order to overcome the guards. Would signs reading 'NO AGGRESSION' have much effect?

An important part of prevention is planning. This is the second stage of the problem-solving process. Thoughtful discussion about preventing possible problems will enable the team to prepare plans for most events. A planned action is far better than a knee-jerk response.

COPING WITH DIFFICULT BEHAVIOUR

Coping is the process of maintaining self – self-esteem, integrity and well-being – in a situation. When used by itself without other strategies it is a short-term measure used by individuals who have little ability to think of long-term issues or of other people, but it is a useful strategy if the individual feels she has little control over her experience. A nurse who is in charge of a ward with half the staff off-sick, and little support or help from her seniors, will cope with it. She will manage to do the things she has to do but will have acquired in the process some negative feelings which may not be easy to get rid of. In very stressful situations we sometimes will sooner panic than cope. In many ways it is the child in us which panics or copes. Burn-out may be the result of stress that has built up over long periods of coping.

DEALING WITH DIFFICULT BEHAVIOUR

Dealing with a situation is a much more parental activity. When a nurse deals with a patient she makes things all right for the patient and when she deals with a difficult situation she is making it all right for the organization. One of the ways nurses are judged by seniors, sometimes unfairly, is by the amount of difficulties that they are perceived as having. If a nurse deals with difficulties and does not report them she may well be seen in a positive light but a nurse who correctly makes it known to her senior that there are problems in her area of responsibility may be judged as someone who has difficulties or even as someone who is difficult.

Quite clearly, protecting seniors from difficulties in this way is immoral and unprofessional. It prevents appropriate solutions from being found for difficulties. A common event in the health service, as in most organizations, is for the recipient of a complaint to hold the view that it's not her fault and then to fail to pass the complaint on. It is rare for any senior nurse to know of all occasions on which patients make threatening remarks to the staff. It would be interesting to know how many nurses in an out-patients' department fail to pass on remarks made about doctors by waiting patients. The nurses who simply deals with everything may be showing some professional skills but is preventing the natural development of the service.

Used in isolation prevention of, coping with and dealing with difficult behaviour are generally ineffective and a waste of organizational and personal resources. However, when used in combination they do begin to have an effect. A good example of this is teaching self-defence to nurses. In isolation it would be of little use and could even be a danger. As a side-effect it may be that the nurse will feel more confident and therefore behave in a more appropriate manner, but without other resources (personal, organizational and practical) the training will be wasted.

If prevention, coping and dealing are combined with an adult approach they become management.

MANAGING AGGRESSION

Managing aggression is about being thoughtful, deliberate and, most important of all, about being active. It is far better to have tried to do something which turned out badly than not to have bothered doing anything. Of course sometimes the nurse may take an active decision to 'do nothing', that is to wait, observe or to allow someone else to act. Management includes creating short- and long-term goals, recognizing the needs of the patient, of the nurse, of other people and of the organization and acknowledging the individuality and the rights of those involved.

Frustration and boredom are two identified causes of aggression and violence. Anyone who has had to attend an out-patients' or casualty department on more than one occasion will have experience of this. By taking an active approach the nurses can reduce these factors to a minimum. Those who merely cope or deal with this tend to struggle on, feeling disenchanted and becoming frustrated and bored themselves.

An active manager is able to identify the problems, plan a course of action, realize those plans and then evaluate the results. This is problem-solving, the central process in good nursing; it is the nursing process. Nurses have learned to use this approach when dealing with an individual patient but as a group they have in general failed to value it as an overall strategy for less specific problems and as a very rewarding way of managing their managers.

Often the approach to the problems associated with difficult patients is erratic and piecemeal. As an example many patients and relatives spend an inordinate amount of time waiting in an A&E department (Royal Commission 1978; Raphael and Handeville 1977; Sadler 1988) and this can be a major contribution to difficult behaviour. Many nurses cope with the difficult patient by being 'philosophical' (a word which is given a meaning completely opposite to its real one) and by moaning to each other or to their friends. Some nurses deal with situations by being autocratic and distant and may react with anger to the patient's anger. Some organizations advocate higher security, while others display health education posters. The two last approaches may be accompanied by meetings with more noise being generated, more hours being worked and more money being spent but they do not by themselves result in much being done. On the other hand nurses taking an active approach are able to have an impact on the conditions under which they work (Dunn 1988).

SUMMARY

Most difficult behaviour can be described using five categories: withdrawal, passivity, manipulation, aggression and violence. In order to become effective the nurse needs to combine prevention of, coping with and dealing with difficult behaviour with an adult approach. The qualities of the adult approach include respect, empathy and genuineness. These are central to the effective management of other people. In managing difficult behaviour they are essential.

7 Managing the Environment

A FRIENDLY PLACE

The environment in which the patient is encountered is an important aspect of managing aggression and violence and it ought to be easy to change and develop. For instance, the effort required to make seating more comfortable for the patients should be less than that which is required to help the staff to be better communicators. In the modern health service, as with most large organizations, this is not so. For the professional person, the process of acquiring suitable equipment and support services can be frustrating and confusing.

The kind of things which can make the environment more helpful when managing aggression are those which relieve boredom, reduce uncertainty and anxiety, increase comfort and lead to people having more respect for the organization and those in it. Lack of them affects the quality of the patient's visit to hospital and that of the nurse's working life. Therefore the nurse – and especially the nurse in charge – has a duty to attempt to overcome the obstacles in the system. The first choice of action must be to use adult skills to explain the situation to seniors and bring pressure to bear in an attempt to have the situation resolved. Where the situation is a threat to the well-being of people there is an additional need to act. This must be accompanied by fulfilling such administrative needs as the completion of 'hazard reports' or otherwise reporting to a health and safety representative.

Two of the places in which the patients might experience the greatest difficulties is in out-patients' and A&E departments. These two places represent the two extremes of the service that the NHS provides. In out-patients' the patients are adults who have come along for an appointment to discuss a non-urgent problem. There is a certain inevitability about an out-patient's visit. The department almost always seems peripheral to the rest of the hospital; it is cold and colourless with uncomfortable and cramped seating. Information is hard to come by and the staff are distant and unknown. The whole department is doctor-centred. The patients are seen as an irritation that can interfere with the smooth functioning of the department.

On the other hand in the A&E department the patients are often in the child position. They are hurt, confused and insecure. However mild their problem, it feels urgent and sometimes life-threatening. There are generally no appointments and waiting time is therefore unpredictable. The hospital seems to centre around the department with lots of very clever and busy staff dealing with all kinds of important problems. Information is hard to come by and seating is uncomfortable. While the A&E department is more patient-centred it is still easy for the patient to feel left out of things.

Even where this is not so it may often seem to be true to the waiting patient. It is part of the nurse's responsibility to make these departments feel different. Ideally the patients should experience the department as a friendly place where the experts have the time and the skills to make them feel welcomed and cared for. Information should be readily available and patients should feel that the place is run by competent and efficient people.

Boredom

This can be a major cause of aggression. Boredom will lead to the patients having little else to do but contemplate their feelings and situation. Any feelings contributing to aggression will begin to assume disproportionate importance. A similar process can take place with pain. A toothache which has been mildly distracting during a busy day can become overwhelming at night. During the day the pain is competing with other stimuli but when the sufferer has settled down for the night the pain becomes the major stimulus and therefore seems much greater. Distraction will diminish the pain. This principle applies to all sources of discomfort and stress. Where a patient has little to distract him from his difficulties his frustration and anger will become the major source of emotional stimulus.

The distraction is only needed where there is the opportunity for boredom. Shorter waiting periods would prevent the problem arising most of the time. For an account of patients' feelings about this and other matters see the Royal Commission (1978) report. Of course the nurse may have little control over the level of activity in her department, especially where that activity is unpredictable and where other non-nursing staff are particularly independent. The nurse must also be aware that different people will have different thresholds of boredom. A resourceful person who feels unstressed, is not too worried and with no alternative demands on their time will have little trouble waiting. Another, who has few resources, is worried and rushed, will find almost any delay intolerable.

The distraction must also be relevant to the waiting person. Health care posters, although they are displayed with the best intention, are usually an insult to the waiting patient. Imagine the irony of coming to hospital with chest pains or with a relative who has been in a road accident and enduring an inordinate wait in the A&E department while all around you are posters telling you to brush your teeth, eat plenty of fibre and not to drink and drive. These are ridiculously irrelevant and will exaggerate the patient's feelings rather than distract him from them. It is difficult to provide suitable distraction to someone who is undergoing great physical trauma but the greater the trauma the less the patient or relative should be kept waiting. In an outpatients' or A&E department waiting area there ought to be the opportunity either to sit quietly or to watch television/video. Anyone who is so upset that television would upset them further should not be left sitting in a communal waiting area.

Children's boredom can be relieved by the provision of safe and good quality toys. Many clinics and departments have old damaged toys. Toys would also reduce the stress inflicted upon parents and others by the disruption caused by bored children.

Uncertainty

Uncertainty is a major cause of stress. Possibility of bad news can be harder to deal with than the bad news itself and the anxiety of waiting is very often far greater than the anxiety of finding out. This is because imagination of what is wrong is usually far worse than reality. Once a person knows the difficulties they are facing it is easier for them to take the steps needed to come to terms with them and to make the necessary adjustments to their lives. If the nurse is skilled at keeping a patient informed it is far better to give them as much information as possible even when something is likely but not definite.

This applies to what, for nurses, might be quite basic information. If the waiting patient is unsure how long they will have to wait the wait will seem interminable. Thus even a wait of forty-five minutes becomes stressful and even intolerable. If the patient knows the wait will be for two hours and that there is a good reason for this, and a good reason why they can't go and come back later, then they will, by and large, wait peacefully for two hours or more. An accurate and understandable electronic display indicating waiting time is probably the single most important practical measure that can be taken to reduce conflict between patients and staff in the A&E department. There is no excuse to not have one. Such organizations as British Rail, London Underground and British Airports Authority have recognized this. Giving a quick shout into the waiting room (Bradley 1984) is neither enough nor very reassuring. The system needs to be well-presented and reliable and used to enhance interactions rather than a substitute for them.

Anxiety may not always present as expected. Someone who is wringing his hands or crying may be identified as worried or concerned but a person who is shouting and threatening is not likely to be seen as anxious. People tend to view displays of weakness as anxiety while exhibitions of strength rarely are. If I took my sick or injured child to a surgery or hospital and experienced undue delay I would become demanding. Besides my belief that I have a duty to obtain the very best for my children I would feel anxious. I would be more likely to express that anxiety in a way I thought would not only reduce the anxiety but also get some results. I would become very demanding and obstinate.

It is important to realize that preventing unnecessary anxiety will make all patients (and staff) more cooperative and relaxed. It is also good practice to try and reassure those who are being aggressive or violent. When a good psychiatric nurse restrains a violent patient he or she tells the patient that the nurses will not hurt him, that things are all right and makes sure that the patient is aware of what will happen. The effect on even the most uncontrolled patient is quite noticeable. Reassurance need not always be verbal. The simple act of staying calm will often reduce another person's anxiety. It is the greatest failing of many nurses that when confronted by an excited patient they become excited. In the same way that an excited patient provokes excitation in the nurse an excited nurse will aggravate an uncontrolled patient.

Perhaps the best way for the nurse to calm someone is for her to feel like and behave like an adult. An adult environment will also have this calming effect.

AN ADULT ENVIRONMENT

The adult environment is one which demonstrates that the people in it respect each other. A neglected or grubby department or ward will convey a number of messages. It will suggest that 'the powers which be', whoever they are, have little respect for the staff working there; that these staff must therefore be unimportant and in some respects subservient. The patient's need for the service offered may only confuse the issue. A patient may have difficulty in understanding his own position and that of others in a hierarchy. One of the ways of resolving a conflict about someone's place in a hierarchy is by testing and a patient who is unclear about the roles and authority of nurses might do this by trying to put the nurses 'in their place'.

Another message that can be conveyed by neglected surroundings is that the customer is not important. Organizations which value their customers spend a lot of time and money making them feel valued. Part of this is expressed in the surroundings which the customer encounters. Organizations which wish to discourage the customer's presence deliberately try to put them off. A good way to do this is to avoid spending money on decoration, furniture and maintenance. Prisons, DSS offices and visa departments are examples. Quite clearly many health service departments are more like social security offices than places where the customer is respected and cared for.

Respect is one of three qualities which must be present in all good nursing practice. The others are empathy and genuineness. A well-presented environment will convey all of these, assuming that the staff live up to the patient's raised expectations. A patient who sees staff who are valued and respected and who feels he is valued and respected will cooperate with the organization and use less time and fewer resources. Aggression and violence are less likely to occur in a well-maintained environment.

A part of making the patient feel respected is to offer him a degree of comfort. This will also serve to help the patient settle while waiting and arouse less frustration. A health service with a responsibility to encourage health and well-being must consider the effects of poor seating on patients and staff. Failure to provide comfortable and safe seating is negligence. Although it seems difficult to justify anything but a sympathetic approach to patient care this is often not evident. Making a patient's visit or stay comfortable is in the interests of both the staff and the patient.

Balanced Security

While it is possible to create an environment which helps with the management of aggression (DHSS 1975) it is impossible to prevent it altogether. The amount of contact potentially aggressive patients have with staff can be reduced. Reinforced glass will protect a nurse from almost all assaults but it does not contribute to the comfortable, secure and welcoming environment needed to help prevent aggression. Similarly use of guards may in the long term increase the level of aggression. Security measures must be discreet. They have limited deterrent value and are often provocative.

Many secure wards protect their television by enclosing it in a plywood box so that it is inaccessible to anyone without a key. Clearly televisions do need protecting from uncontrolled patients because they make very effective weapons. However enclosing them in cheap undecorated plywood boxes may make them a focus of aggression. In the same way that subservient behaviour may be an invitation to be treated badly so might a wooden box protecting the television be an invitation to be aggressive or violent towards it. Pointing out that this is a vulnerable area may focus attention on it. Some wards accept that occasionally the television will be destroyed, do not enclose it but secure it to prevent it being used as a missile. Generally on such wards there is a greater respect for the patient's individuality and the ward is more often a brighter and more attractive place. These are the wards which tend to have less aggression and violence.

Anything which distances the staff from the patient and makes the patient feel hard done by is contributing to the level of aggression of the patients and inflicted upon the staff. Security measures must be kind to be effective.

The easiest way to make security kind is to operate a system which is able to respond to difficult situations. Where there is a need it is better to have a call team available to assist rather than use indiscriminate security. The team should not consist just of large males. It should include someone with both innate and appointed authority – an assertive manager – and it should include female as well as male staff. Aggressive men especially can respond much more positively to a woman. A man may be seen as more of a threat or a more acceptable victim. Such a team must comprise mostly nurses because not only will they have a more professional approach but will be trained to communicate, have experience of interacting with a wide variety of people and be familiar with many of the administrative processes involved. Additionally nurses generally have the most balanced approach. They have the approach of the professional and like the doctors, psychologists, OTs and managers have an understanding of the organization, themselves and of the needs of the patients. They have an essentially practical experience of their work which covers a very broad spectrum of care and responsibility. The ideal team would consist of male and female nurses with both RMN and RGN qualifications and of several grades. In places where there is much aggression and violence as well as other difficult behaviour it is prudent to employ a suitable qualified psychiatric nurse in a specialist role. This nurse would be able to assist, educate and advise other staff. There should be aggression management nurses just as there are occupational health and infection control nurses, and health authorities should consider creating them.

Where there is a need to call other staff to assist with aggressive incidents there must be an easily used and reliable call system. The telephone is useless unless there is a special alarm included in the system. A press button system is far safer and although there are more likely to be false alarms these can serve as practice.

When considering the level of security to be provided it is important to look at the layout of a ward or department. There should be nowhere for an assailant to corner staff and isolate them from escape or help. It is essential that areas where those at risk work or are treated are open to general observation. Doors should swing open and not shut when left; bed curtains should always be left drawn back when not needed. When difficult patients, or even those who are suspected of being difficult, are seen there should be a second person in support or close at hand. Potential weapons should be reduced to a minimum. As is good nursing practice everywhere, sharp instruments should be safely stored and safely disposed of. Where there is any suspicion a search should be made of the patient's clothing and property. This might be overt or discreet depending on the skills of the staff and the nature of the patient. If visitors are thought to be a threat they should be asked to wait in the waiting area, assuming that all the above advice has been followed.

SUMMARY

The environment should be comfortable and friendly and convey the message to the staff and the patients that they are valued and respected. Where there is unavoidable waiting time there should be a variety of distractions and facilities. Information about all aspects of the patient's visit should be readily available.

A secure environment has good lighting and visibility with no places to hide. Dangerous items and those with any value to a potential thief should be securely locked away. There will be an easily used alarm system for rapidly summoning skilled help. It will also be a place where attention to health and safety considerations have meant that, for instance, falling is less dangerous.

8 Being Adult

To be an effective approach 'adultness' must become part of the nurse's personality. How it is used will depend on her role but it is not something she can pretend to do. The nurse must think, feel and behave like an adult to have the desired effect on others.

It is vitally important that the adultness is conveyed to others, that certain something which lets others know that the nurse is responsible, objective, reliable and fair. There are a number of things she can do to help demonstrate her maturity. Most of the strategies described below will not only demonstrate adultness but will enhance it. The best way to become more adult is to practise.

The important elements involved in presenting adultness are the spoken language, non-verbal communication and eye contact.

THE SPOKEN LANGUAGE

While the spoken word forms the usual method of communication between people it is by no means essential. Some people will not speak, some cannot and some are able to use other ways more effectively. Verbal communication is simply the primary means for most people. For others the primary means may be sign language and for others writing. In order to convey 'adultness' when speaking to a patient the nurse needs to sound confident, clear and concise. Many 'sub-verbal' signs such as stuttering, pausing too much or not enough, tutting and sighing can have a negative effect.

Normal social activity in conversation needs to be developed to a greater level of skill. Most people are able to use techniques such as interruption and questioning. The professional communicator will develop her skills, and be able to use them in a deliberate way.

Interrupting another is not polite in most social situations. If a

patient is having difficulty in expressing an emotion or idea interruption may be enough to make him give up. What is just bad
manners becomes anti-productive when caring for or managing
others. The nurse needs to be very much more aware of the cues in
the conversations of others which allow her to anticipate and plan
her behaviour. However there may be times when it is important for
the nurse to interrupt. She needs to be able to do this in an adult
manner.

Questioning (Niven 1989) is an area at which everyone has some
practice but at which few are accomplished. There are two types of
question, 'open' and 'closed'. An open question is one which leaves
the extent and direction of the response open to the responder. A
closed question restricts the possible answers. 'How do you feel
today?' is an open question. 'Are you all right today?' is a closed
question. Generally questions requiring a 'yes' or 'no', answer are
closed although sometimes open questions are phrased as if they
were closed. 'Can I do anything to help you?' can have a 'yes' or 'no'
answer but the expectation is that the answer will be more involved
such as 'No, thank you, I have managed to . . .'

Open questions are best when it is important to gather com-
plicated or new information and when it is intended for a person to
express themselves in some way. Open questions lead to longer and
more open answers and also help convey a sympathetic and understanding approach. Closed questions are best used when a little
amount of information is needed quickly. They are business-like
and tend to be impersonal.

Sometimes instructions are disguised as questions, as in an
exchange I witnessed:

Sister: 'Would you like to go and collect John from the day
hospital?'
Student: 'No.'

The student treated the sister's instruction as if it was a question
and responded inappropriately. The sister meant 'Go and collect
John.' Much of the time this disguise helps social interactions but at
times may be misinterpreted. On several occasions I have said to

people, 'If I were you I would ... ' and had my comment treated as an instruction. All the respondents who thought that I was being bossy were from other cultures (mostly European). It may well be that there are many such social expressions which lose part of their meaning or gather additional meaning when used with people of different cultural experience. As managers of others, nurses must be wary of this.

NON-VERBAL COMMUNICATION

In a gross sense it is possible to make interpretations about the mental activity of others from their physical activity. It is reasonable to suppose that if a patient is crying, he is unhappy; if he is smiling, he is happy. Language is an aspect of behaviour which is used a great deal in this respect. If a patient tells a nurse that he is frightened of surgery then the nurse can reliably believe him. If a patient says that he will hit the nurse if ... then she best beware of him. What remains a point of disagreement is how far interpretation of non-verbal communication can be taken. Non-verbal communication includes a person's posture and expression.

A skilled person can predict general behaviour from posture and movement. It would be wrong though to believe that it is possible to describe reliably the mental processes involved in another person's behaviour.

Sometimes a nurse may have the impression that a patient is in a particular state. These intuitions should not be dismissed out of hand. During the first stage of the nursing process the possibility that this feeling may have some validity should be considered. The process of gathering information about the patient may be subconscious. Human behaviour is so complex that it is sometimes difficult to describe how it has been perceived and understood.

Nurses should be very wary of the judgements they make of other people's behaviour. It is possible to describe the behaviour of others but it is very much harder to describe the mental processes that give rise to that behaviour. While acknowledging that on occasions we can make accurate assumptions about others, it must be remembered that they are only assumptions.

Sitting posture is a good example. Traditionally a slouched posture suggests disinterest, an upright posture interest and leaning forwards suggests dominance. This may sometimes be true but it is not the only possible explanation of each posture. It may be more comfortable to adopt a particular posture in a certain chair. In dining chairs and in classroom chairs I find it very much more comfortable to slouch as most other positions give me backache after a short while. Those who believe in a fundamental approach to interpretation might suggest that describing physical comfort is a way of describing mental comfort. In other words when I say it is more comfortable to slouch in my chair I am giving a deeper message that it is mentally more comfortable for me. Again this may at times be true.

There is no one who knows enough about me to be able to make this kind of judgement reliably as to be able to use it professionally. After living with and knowing me for many years my parents, siblings, spouse and offspring may become quite good at it. A nurse will very rarely have this level of knowledge about others, especially about a patient she has known for a relatively short time.

The problem for such people as nurses is that other people will interpret their behaviour. A nurse who frowns because she is puzzled may well find that the patient interprets the frowning behaviour as crossness. In order to overcome this danger of misinterpretation the nurse needs to become skilled at presenting what are known as the open positions.

THE OPEN POSITIONS

The open positions are those which demonstrate openness to another person. The closed positions are those in which the body is closed off or defended from others. The open positions give fewer messages for others to misinterpret thus giving greater weight to verbal messages. There are two basic open positions, the seated and the standing. The open seated position is illustrated in Figure 8.1 and the open standing position in Figure 8.2.

Figure 8.1 The open seated position	*Figure 8.2* The open standing position
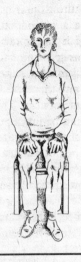	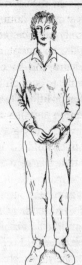

Two problems of the open positions are that they can feel both artificial and uncomfortable. This is especially so for the nurse on the general ward where the patient may well be bedridden. Almost any bedside position is uncomfortable and it is one of the advantages of a more liberal style of ward management that nurses are allowed to sit on the bed when conversing with a patient.

It is all right to modify the above positions so that they feel comfortable and natural. What must be remembered though is that the more they are modified the more liable they are to misinterpretation. To modify the sitting position by crossing one leg over the other and turning the body by 45° is to change from the open to the closed position, giving a message of defensiveness or disinterest. Interlocking fingers is a more realistic modification.

During an aggressive confrontation the act of sitting down can help to calm the situation. The seated nurse can be less threatening and give the message that she is calm. It is also more difficult for someone to attack another person if both are seated side by side.

The major problem with the open standing position is what to do with one's hands. Almost every comfortable position moves away from being open. Hands behind the back, on the hips or folding arms can seem very authoritarian and judgemental. Raising the arms above the shoulder suggests anxiety while clasping the hands in front of the body may have the effect of focusing an aggressive patient's attention on a particular part of the body. The most appropriate modification of the open position is to hold the hands centrally in front of the body. The problem remains however of what to do with them. Almost all activity will convey a message of anxiety or unsureness. The best solution is to hold an appropriate item such as a pen or a piece of paper. Nurses are at an advantage here in that they often have suitable props available to them. Of course a pen can be used as a weapon against the nurse, but this is an unlikely event and in any case a pen is easy to drop should the patient move to attack you. An instrument like a pair of scissors is not suitable.

A nurse who feels confident will convey her feelings by standing firmly. If she hops from one foot to the other, however subtly, the patient will feel that the nurse is unsure of herself.

When nervous energy builds up in the body an individual begins to feel a need to act. When unable to act, as perhaps when a nurse may have to stay and face a situation without much activity, the energy will be channelled into 'displacement activity' or fidgeting. This presents itself as restlessness, foot tapping, fiddling with odds and ends or nattering too much. At times this activity is more socially acceptable than at others. Pens, cigarettes or chewing gum are used to channel the displaced energy. An important part of an open position is that there is no displacement activity.

To some extent the mere absence of negative messages may suggest positive ones. But when it becomes a habit to adopt an open position it will help the nurse to be more relaxed and begin to convey some positive messages. These messages are that the open person is relaxed, secure, calm and attentive. Open positions convey 'adultness'. Other factors such as appropriate distance from others and choosing a suitable place can be used to enhance the interaction.

There is a third 'position' which can be described as 'open' although not traditionally so. This is the 'open' walk. Research some years ago showed that mugging victims tended to walk in a particular way. This included such characteristics as lowered gaze and chin, stooped shoulders, little or poor coordination of arm swing and shorter rapid steps. These people walk like 'little' and unimportant people. The other extreme is to stride along with chin held high and an exaggerated arm swing. The intermediate position is to walk at a moderate pace looking ahead, observing the world like a 'big' person. It is this intermediate position which is the equivalent of the open position conveying a few positive messages. People who walk like this are far less likely to get mugged. When walking about her duties the nurse should be upright and definite. If she communicates her confidence the patients will have more confidence in her and will soon become more confident themselves. This will help them to become more active in their recovery.

EYE CONTACT

There are two extreme things the nurse can do with her eyes when interacting. She can stare into the other person's eyes or can avoid their gaze altogether. Both of these are strange ways to behave in our culture. There are those who advocate a stare claiming that if we look into another's eyes we will be more able to anticipate his actions. It seems a very provocative thing to do and is more likely to lead to an attack of some kind.

On the other hand some experts advise that when interacting with an aggressive patient it is best to look at a point in the middle of his or her sternum (Moran 1984). This is bad and ill-informed advice for two reasons: first, a female will (rightly) assume the nurse is looking at her cleavage and may well misinterpret the nurse's intent; second, the nurse may give the message that she is subservient to the other person. This will on occasions amount to granting permission for the assailant to be violent.

Humans have a natural and occasionally healthy tendency to behave in a hierarchical manner. This serves many important social functions and helps the individual fit into society. However when interacting with a patient (or senior nurse or doctor) in an adult manner it is important that the nurse conveys a sense of equality, that both parties are important with their own needs and own point of view.

When being dominant people will tend to look down on others by doing such things as choosing higher chairs, even raising their chin so that they are able to look down their nose at others. This may be extremely provocative to the patient and may well precipitate an attack. Likewise if the nurse feels dominated she will tend to look down and sometimes away. When she does this she may in effect be giving the patient permission to be dominant. This dominance may for some people include the right to attack the subservient individual. For an excellent account of this kind of behaviour in chimpanzees read *In the Shadow of Man* (van Larwick 1974). We seem to be very like them in our behaviour and the description of the chimpanzee society is a reflection of our own.

The appropriate behaviour again lies between the extremes of staring into the other's eyes or avoiding them and the best approach can be described as face-to-face contact rather than eye-to-eye contact. This is illustrated by tracing the eye movements of a person looking at a picture of a face. Attention generally concentrates around the eyes but includes all the features of the face and the head. This trace forms a very definite impression of a human face (Atkinson *et al*. 1983; Yarbus 1967).

What happens in the face is as important as what happens in the eyes. An open face makes no strong expression, although there must be some spontaneity. It is important to nod to encourage the other to continue the interaction. Nodding is such a powerful tool that even a movement of a few millimetres can have an effect on another's behaviour. A good general rule is that all other things being equal nodding will lead to a behaviour becoming more frequent. Nodding conveys interest, attention and understanding. Other facial activity may convey less positive messages. Frowning, yawning, looking puzzled, confused or distracted are all activities which may help a patient to feel unsure, dissatisfied or frustrated.

The nurse needs to be aware of her own facial expressions and to develop these in a skilled way. Some people have a tendency to smile when nervous or threatened. Some people frown when they are puzzled by something. How does an observer know if the smile indicates amusement, sympathy or nervousness? How many patients who have told a nurse some personal detail will understand that the nurse is puzzled that she has been chosen for this confidence rather than that she is angry?

SUMMARY

There are three main aspects to the way the nurse can present herself as adult. These are the way she uses the spoken language, the way she sits, stands and walks and the way she looks at the person she is talking to. When a nurse has deliberate control over posture, facial contact and language she becomes an effective communicator able to be understood and to understand. An essential tool in managing difficult behaviour is open communication. As soon as a nurse begins to close her means of communication she begins to distance herself from the patient.

9 Physical Responses

However skilled a nurse becomes and whatever measures are taken to provide a good environment there will still, inevitably, be times when violence occurs. When this happens it is important to continue to use an adult assertive approach even though this becomes very much more difficult. There may also be times when it becomes necessary to use physical measures to help manage a person who is not violent. Perhaps a patient is so provocative or otherwise disturbed that they need to be isolated or need to be removed from a particular place. Whatever the justification and however skilled the nurse, many patients who are restrained or isolated view this restraint as an attack.

There may in extreme situations be justification for the nurse to attack or eject the patient. A nurse may be justified in attacking a patient when it appears that not to do so would result in great danger or harm to the nurse or another individual. If for example a nurse walked into a side room on her ward and found a person in the act of throttling another and the assailant continued in spite of the nurse's efforts to pull him away there might then be justification for striking the assailant. It would be most unusual although not impossible for a nurse to encounter such a situation. The same may be true of patients who are ejected from a place where they have been causing difficulties. Occasionally patients refuse to leave the hospital when discharged or to leave a room to allow other patients to be cared for. There then exists a responsibility for someone, perhaps the unit manager or the nurse in charge to take steps to have this person removed so that the hospital can continue with its work. Generally such situations will allow time for assistance to be summoned. It will be possible to call for and await the arrival of security staff or the police.

Physical response can be of several different kinds. It may be restraint, seclusion, self-defence or medication. These are the courses open to most nurses most of the time.

RESTRAINT

Restraint is the more usual form of dealing with violence and ought to follow the guidelines issued by the DoH or the various trade unions and professional organizations. It is important that guidelines are written, widely circulated and universally understood. They are effective only if there is some common understanding of the action to be taken. The most effective techniques are those known as Control and Restraint (C&R) (Needham 1987). This is a set of techniques developed by the Home Office for use in the prison service. It has two main aims, to allow a team of three nurses effectively to restrain an aggressive patient and to allow a victim to break away from her assailant. There is a third aim which is generally not applicable to NHS staff and is that of riot control. Given that an organized and proven method of restraint is available employers are obliged by law to make sure that their staff are trained in it. Where there is no local skill in C&R techniques staff must rely on more general recommendations.

SECLUSION

This is a more sophisticated form of restraint and its only purpose must be to protect others from the patient, to protect a patient from himself (including the danger of provoking others) and to isolate the patient from contact which might otherwise cause him to deteriorate. Seclusion must also follow strict guidelines issued by those responsible. A good seclusion policy will allow for the times when staff must act first and then acknowledge procedures. A good seclusion policy can exist in A&E departments and general wards where there might be occasion to isolate patients for psychiatric reasons.

SELF-DEFENCE

This is different from restraint and seclusion in that it is not carried out in the patient's interest. A patient can be restrained or secluded only when there is an adequate number of staff available. When one nurse finds herself alone and under attack and unable to escape she must act to protect herself. If she has adopted an adult approach and failed to dissuade her assailant she must then consider using force to defend herself. There are three ways to defend oneself: first, to fight tooth and nail, struggling with the attacker; second, to use a recognized and learned system of self-defence – judo, karate, etc; and third, to use the established breakaway techniques as a means of escape.

The disadvantage of the first is that such an unskilled defence will usually fail. It may also provoke the attacker into a more violent act in order to overcome the defence or because of greater anger. Learning a recognized system of self-defence is ideal but for most nurses impractical. It is certainly unrealistic to expect the health service to provide such a training for all nurses. The amount of time and money needed would be prohibitive and the effectiveness would anyway be diminished by the volume of learners. Where a nurse is able to make use of local facilities then this would be advisable. Health authorities ought to make some effort to provide such training only when they have addressed more effective courses of action associated with prevention and breakaway techniques which can be more economically taught.

What must be well understood and cannot be emphasized enough is that using a book to learn self-defence is a grave mistake. Like all motor skills self-defence must be taught by a skilled person and practised and developed with their help. Someone who has taught themselves from a book and without the help of a trained instructor is in great danger because of the false sense of security they will have and the lack of reliable feedback on their progress.

The most sensible approach is to use 'breakaway techniques'. These are simple responses to an attack developed by the Home Office and aimed at allowing a victim quickly to escape an attacker.

They can be easily learned by groups of nurses in a comparatively short time and when practised are most effective. They enable the victim to take the most sensible course when attacked – to escape.

MEDICATION

When giving medication to control an aggressive or violent patient a nurse should remember a number of things in addition to the usual conventions and codes.

First, medication is a treatment for an illness. It is not a means of restraining a criminal. It can only be given for therapeutic reasons. If given for reasons which are not therapeutic the act of injection might constitute assault.

Second, most medication which will control aggression takes some time to act even if given intra-muscularly. About half an hour should be allowed. Care must be taken not to give medication to the patient every ten minutes on the assumption that the previous dose was ineffective. Any additional support to manage the patient should be arranged for and retained for at least half an hour. Some tranquillizers can be given intravenously and are therefore usually (but not always) very much more effective. There is still the danger of topping up too quickly. Most of the 'major tranquillizers' can have horrendous side-effects which usually become worse with higher doses although not all are dose-related.

Third, suitable medication should be prescribed 'as needed' when the major tranquillizers are prescribed for the first time or given to new patients.

Fourth, and finally, giving intra-muscular medication to a struggling patient is a risky business. There is an increased danger of needle-stick injury. It is not unknown for the injecting nurse to inject a fellow nurse's leg in mistake for the patient's. There is also the risk of damaging the patient as he struggles. Whenever possible an experienced nurse should give the injection and there should be adequate staff safely to restrain the patient without inflicting pain or injury.

A most effective medicine for helping to gain control of someone in an emergency is Paraldehyde. While this is out of fashion because it has no anti-psychotic effect it is very effective as a sedative and is far safer than other 'tranquillizers'. Its side-effects are fewer and less frightening for the patient than the more commonly used drugs and it can give the patient greatly needed relief and respite.

SUMMARY

Whatever the nurse is able to do there will be times when she needs to resort to physical measures to manage aggression. These can take the form of restraint, seclusion, self-defence or medication. The Home Office-developed system of Control and Restraint is designed to allow the nurse to contain an aggressive situation. Medication can also be used to help the patient settle but should not be used just as a means of control.

10 Forming a Policy

In forming or reviewing a general policy for managing aggression it is best to consider all the factors to ensure a balanced and comprehensive approach. Such a review should include:

(a) The general philosophy of the health authority/unit and specific considerations like staff support,
> training,
> health and safety,
> service provision, and
> systems of review.
(b) Psychological methods.
(c) Self-defence.
(d) Restraint.
(e) Seclusion.

Due consideration must be given to the 1983 Mental Health Act (Jones 1985). Where they have access to a psychiatrist and perhaps to a mental health nurse there is no reason why general hospitals and especially A&E departments should not have secure or seclusion rooms. A good secure room is purpose-built or adapted. It is reserved only for that use being free of all items except a bed and having reinforced fittings and no place for the patient to cut or to hang himself.

The general philosophy and the specific considerations should be developed by the appropriate practitioners. There is a tendency for groups looking at such policies to use senior managers, doctors and senior nurses. See, for instance, the membership of the Lord Skelmersdale committee (DHSS, 1989). It is invariably ward and community nurses who manage the aggression and violence and who have the expertise. It is essential to include an educationalist in the development of such policies as they are able to offer the special skills and understanding unique to the educational process involved in implementing the policy.

Self-defence must be formally taught to be effective. Formal training must be provided or staff encouraged to seek their own training. Whatever the decision it must be remembered that limited resources might best be directed to preventive measures – both environmental and educational. The authority must state its policy concerning staff who have found it necessary to defend themselves and should take account of and describe the legal position of its employees.

INITIAL ACTION

Prevention must be the primary objective of all staff. It is recognized however that on occasions prevention will not be possible.

When a patient begins to behave in an aggressive or violent manner the nurse present (the responsible nurse) should attempt to:

(1) Adopt an open position.
(2) Remain calm, be objective and as non-threatening as possible.
(3) Continue to talk to and listen to the patient, being as reassuring as possible, unless the patient finds it aggravating.
(4) Make no false promises and tell no lies to the patient.
(5) Place themselves in a position which allows them to escape if need be.
(6) Summon help if this can be done without antagonizing the patient.
(7) Prevent others from threatening the patient.

Staff going to the assistance (assisting nurses) of a nurse managing a potentially violent patient should:

(8) While taking care not to delay, approach the situation calmly and without rushing and threatening the patient.
(9) Remove items likely to cause injury – watches, pens, glasses and ties – out of sight of the patient.

(10) Observe the situation they find and decide whether it is best to wait out of sight, in sight of either the responsible nurse or the patient or both or to take over.

(11) If time allows, remove other patients, visitors, etc. from the scene.

Staff must be patient in attempting to resolve an aggressive situation. They should attempt to negotiate an end rather than force it upon others. They must also have regard to the idea of boundary-setting – that some people respond well and/or need to have the boundaries of acceptable behaviour defined for them. Sometimes prolonged negotiation can be seen as a sign of weakness which the patient feels he can exploit. Being firm is an important part of negotiation as is having a 'bottom line' – a point at which the negotiation has to stop and action be taken. Understanding the institution's and her own boundaries will help both the nurse and the patient operate within them.

(12) When the situation begins to become calmer the assisting nurses should withdraw a little. When the situation is resolved key personnel should remain available, out of sight but within hailing distance or perhaps sitting with other patients presenting themselves as a model of calmness.

(13) Even where the situation has been resolved without incident a full report should be made in the patient's nursing notes, in the medical notes via the medical members of the team and on the appropriate incident and/or hazard reports.

(14) Staff should discuss the situation and be allowed to ventilate their feelings and allowed some time to be by themselves.

(15) Normal relationships should be resumed with the patient as soon as possible with as little fuss as possible.

Where attempts to calm the situation fail and it becomes necessary to use physical intervention the priorities must be:

(a) for the nurse to remain in a state which allows her to carry out her functions,

(b) to protect the safety and well-being of third parties, and

(c) to protect the safety and well-being of the aggressor.

It is important that the nurse takes care of her own safety so that she can continue to influence the situation and help to resolve it.

(16) When acts of violence occur the nurse must where practical leave the patient until there is a sufficient number of staff to restrain him.

(17) If defending herself the nurse should use recognized techniques (Needham 1987) and attempt to flee safely.

(18) Where this is not possible and the nurse's life or well-being is threatened she should attempt to disable the patient temporarily and then escape.

(19) When a patient becomes violent the nurse should if possible continue to talk to him. She should only scream for help when the situation has become very threatening.

(20) If it has been possible for a lone nurse to restrain the patient she should give careful consideration to her ability to escape and to her ability to continue to hold him until help arrives.

(21) Assisting nurses arriving on the scene should act quickly and decisively.

The most effective method of restraining a violent patient is to use C&R techniques (Needham 1987). Where the staff are not trained in these they must follow guidelines laid down for the restraint of violent patients. They must be careful not to inflict unnecessary pain upon the patient and not to use hard objects to assist in restraint as has been erroneously recommended (Bradley 1984). Apart from the nurse's duty not to inflict unnecessary pain, it is a waste of time relying on pain as a means of defence as many aggressive and violent people have an abnormally high pain threshold. Those who have taken alcohol or drugs of abuse, those in a heightened emotional state (e.g. angry or anxious) and some patients suffering from psychotic states can all be expected to tolerate higher levels of pain.

RESTRAINT

(1) Restraint should take place only when there is an adequate number and mix of skilled staff.

(2) The nurse in charge should take responsibility for the patient's head her tasks being to:

   (a) Talk to the patient, reassuring him and explaining what is happening.

   (b) Listen to him so that she knows when he is calming or if he is experiencing undue pain, etc.

   (c) Protect the patient's head and neck from damage due to friction, tension, strangulation and impact.

   (d) Prevent the patient from biting or head-butting.

   (e) Direct the other staff as needed.

She thus becomes the responsible nurse.

(3) The assisting nurses should take hold of the patient's limbs, preferably getting a firm grip on his clothing. They will prevent him from hitting or kicking.

(4) By using their own weight and some leverage they will lower the patient to the floor as gently as is practical.

(5) Once the patient is on the floor the nurses will continue to immobilize him without pain by bringing pressure to to bear on the clothing they hold and onto parts of his body which are not tender or subject to twisting or bending.

(6) The nurses will continue to restrain the patient until he is calm or until there is an adequate number and skill mix to remove him to a more suitable place.

(7) Following such an incident support will be offered to the patient, the nurses involved and others who have witnessed the incident.

(8) Care will be taken to ensure that the patient understands what has happened and what may happen.

(9) All nurses involved will make a written report of the incident and the responsible nurse will ensure that all official forms and records are completed.

Sometimes restraint is not enough and a patient will fail to calm down or desist in the behaviour which led to the restraint. Where this occurs the possibility of seclusion should be considered. By this time it is likely that senior staff are present. If they are to make the decision they should give due consideration to all factors including the opinions and the feelings of both the patient and the nurses who will have to care for him.

Seclusion (Leopoldt 1985; MIND 1974; Morrison and le Roux 1987; Shepherd and Deregowski 1981) should be used as means of *safely* containing a patient whose behaviour is such that he is a danger to himself, to others and to property and where he cannot desist from being a danger and where the seclusion will provide the patient or others with that safety.

Seclusion can be described in two ways which here will be called seclusion and isolation.

(1) Isolation is the act of isolating (usually forceably) a patient from other people, that is locking them alone in a room.
(2) Seclusion is the act of removing the patient from the presence of other people *other than staff*. A patient held in a room with only nurses, doctors or people assisting them (security staff and police for instance) is being secluded.

Most of the criticism against 'seclusion' is in fact against the practice of isolating patients. Very often what is here described as seclusion is not regarded or recorded as such. It is far safer to regard any separation from other patients as seclusion. It should be used to safeguard the patient and others. Isolation might also be used. Although it is open to more criticism and causes greater ethical dilemmas it has some advantages. There may be times when the continued presence of the staff is provocative and it is impossible to calm a patient but also essential to contain him. There are also some patients especially those who are over-active who may respond very negatively to the excitement of being restrained. The isolation might enable them to become calmer.

Seclusion

(1) Whenever possible the patient should make his own way to seclusion escorted by adequate staff. Where the patient is unable to do this restraint guidelines apply.
(2) The patient should be as clear as is practical about the nature of

seclusion.

(3) A registered nurse must be responsible for overseeing the seclusion throughout and there must be the appropriate mix and numbers of staff present in the seclusion room or immediately to hand outside it.

(4) The patient's views should be taken into account when deciding on the staff to supervise the seclusion and when the seclusion will end.

(5) The seclusion should be as short as possible and there must be guidelines for its regular review – perhaps every half an hour by the nurse in charge, every two hours jointly by nursing and medical representatives of the care team.

(6) The seclusion should be fully documented with all details recorded.

Isolation

(1) Whenever isolation becomes necessary all the above advice still applies.

(2) By the nature of isolation it will be an emergency measure but wide consultation should take place immediately the patient is secure.

(3) A registered nurse should be allocated and available to supervise the isolation.

(4) A nurse should be present outside the door of the room making frequent observation, balancing the need to protect the patient's welfare against the provocative effect of being constantly watched. Observation should be at least every five minutes.

(5) Adequate numbers and mix of staff must be available to go quickly to the patient's aid should the need arise.

(6) Isolation should be reviewed constantly – at each act of observation and on each occasion that it is discussed. It should be as short as possible.

(7) Following isolation the patient should remain under supportive and observational supervision.

(8) Each case of isolation should be fully documented and discussed at the next team meeting.

A record of all acts of aggression and violence should be kept in all the patient's notes and documentation. All hospitals should have a restraint, seclusion and isolation book. These records must be available for Mental Health Act Commissioners, the Community Health Council and any other official body which represents the patient's or the nurse's interests. There should be a regular policy review looking at the incidents over longer periods – perhaps every six months.

While not normally regarding it as seclusion a record should be kept of all occasions on which any door is locked which prevents the normal mobility of any patient.

The DHSS (1989) report *Violence to Staff* gives good guidelines on the format used to report violent and aggressive incidents. While its recommendations recognize the advantages of local adaptation it would seem important to coordinate national figures making standardization of documentation and its use essential. Other documents of interest include Birmingham 1974a and b; DHSS (N. Ireland) 1980; RCN 1987; RCP 1986. Some of these are locally developed guidelines. Most District Health Authorities have their own and it is worth seeking out the local version and comparing it to others.

SUMMARY

When a policy is being developed a wide range of considerations should be included. It should give guidelines covering initial action, restraint, seclusion and isolation. Statements on the organization's policies should be included. Important points are the idea of responsible and assisting nurses and their roles in restraining and the difference between seclusion (the removal of a patient from other patients and visitors) and isolation (the removal of a patient from all other people). The most important consideration must always be the safety of the people involved.

When dealing with the aggressive or violent patient the professional responsibility of the nurse can be described under a number of headings. These are the duty to care (Walsh 1986), reasonable force (Jones 1985), the Code of Conduct (UKCC 1984), health and safety legislation (TUC 1989) and her contractual duty. Like most responsibilities these also involve the rights of the nurse.

These duties do not suddenly appear when the nurse is confronted by an aggressive patient. The nurse's duty includes preparing herself for what can happen.

THE DUTY TO CARE

Like any other worker (and perhaps anyone who gives advice and assistance) a nurse has a duty to take care in carrying out her function (Jones 1982). Her acts must not be of a nature which will lead to the patients being harmed or neglected. If she does cause harm to a patient, or fails to act in the patient's best interest when she could have, she has then failed in her duty.

The nurse's duty to care is also included in the Code of Conduct so the nurse is in effect answerable to two masters in this respect – the law and the UKCC. Most nurses are aware of their obligation to avoid action which will harm the patient. They are often unaware of their duty to act (UKCC 1984).

Some years ago an informal but suicidal psychiatric patient discharged himself from a hospital. No attempt was made to stop him as he was 'informal'. He subsequently attempted suicide, was admitted to another psychiatric hospital and eventually recovered. He later successfully sued the first hospital because he had been allowed to leave and there had been a failure in the duty to care (verbal report 1983). Even when the nurse does not feel supported by specific legislation she still has a duty to act in a way which safeguards her patients, even where the patient may not agree. This will mean that on some occasions she will have to prevent a patient who is not detained under the 1983 Act from leaving the hospital.

To complicate matters it is difficult to define 'patient' as many people are out-patients, just discharged or about to be admitted. The act of admission or discharge does not in itself define 'patient'. Someone who is seeking admission also has the right to expect the nurse to take care as does a relative. The nurse has a general duty to 'society' (UKCC 1984 item 9) and when balancing the patient's right to freedom and her duty to care she must consider the rights of members of the public and those of other patients both actual and future.

REASONABLE FORCE

The rights of the patient and the public may conflict with the nurse's duty to act. The nurse must remember her rights under the Criminal Law Act (1967) section 3(1). A person can use in the prevention of crime or in arresting a suspected offender 'such force as is reasonable'. Reasonable force is the minimum needed to prevent the crime being committed or to effect the arrest (Jones 1985).

This applies when the nurse is a victim of an assault. She is entitled to use reasonable force to protect herself as assault is a crime. If she uses excessive force she may then be guilty of assault. When deciding on reasonable force there are a number of factors to take into account, such as the size and nature of the assailant and that of the victim, the intent of the attacker, the use of weapons and the likelihood of the attack succeeding. The degree to which the victim felt threatened is also important. In law a threat has to be realistic to be considered a threat and it may sometimes be best to ignore unrealistic or silly threats.

In 1988 a nurse working for a south coast health authority was dismissed for striking a patient. She had approached a confused elderly male patient who had been refusing medication. During the exchange the patient slapped her once across the face. She then slapped him across the face, was reported and sacked. The patient had assaulted the nurse. Her response should have been to use the minimum force needed to prevent the attack continuing. The patient did not continue so the nurse's response was also assault. If the patient had launched a prolonged attack and if the nurse had been able to remove herself from danger she had a legal obligation to do so. Fleeing an attacker is using minimal force and where safe it is in law much the preferred option. Had the nurse been held by the patient while he continued to hit her and if she had felt endangered and believed that she must hit him to protect herself she would have then been justified in her response.

In the late 1970s, while giving first-aid to a victim of an assault, I turned to find myself in danger. A patient was about to throw a pot of steaming tea over me. I had four options: (1) to flee, (2) to tell the patient to stop, (3) to attempt to restrain the assailant and (4) to cause the assailant to cease his act. Option 1 was out of the question as this would have left the first victim unprotected. A nurse under these circumstances has a duty to care for both patients. In any case flight may not have removed the danger as sometimes a fleeing victim is as much at risk as if they stay. To tell the patient to stop was in this case unrealistic. Restraint is always the preferred option when using physical strength to intervene. However on this occasion it was probable that it would have led to both the victim and the assailant being burned. The fourth option was the most sensible and to this end I struck the patient a smart blow on the chin. While doing no damage to the patient it caused him to stagger backwards and drop the pot. The patient was then restrained by other nurses arriving on the scene while others gave first-aid to the victim.

This illustrates the difference between self-defence and assault. It also serves to make another point. Most nurses (and other people) believe that the nurse's first duty is to her patient. This is untrue. The nurse's first duty must always be to herself. She has a right to expect reasonable treatment from others and to be free from threat and danger. Also it will be difficult for a nurse to fulfil her duty to care if she is not fit and healthy herself. Lifting is a good example. A nurse who lifts badly may damage her back. She will have time off sick and reduce the nursing time and skills available to patients. Apart from her duty to herself and her family she also has a duty to be available to the patients. This is equally true of the nurse as victim of assault. While fulfilling her duty to care she must make sure she is able to continue that duty.

Only the nurse who is there at the time can balance her duty to care, her duty to look after herself and her duty to society. Her decision unavoidably will be influenced by her personality and her role. As long as she does her best and acts 'in good faith' she will be open to no valid criticism.

To confuse matters someone who is insane is not capable of committing a crime so it becomes difficult under the Criminal Law Act (1967) to use any force to prevent his actions. It would seem though that anyone, and especially someone who has a professional role in the matter, can act as if the person was not insane. For the nurse this is partly because of her duty to care but also because common law allows an individual to use reasonable force in self-defence and in the defence of others.

PROFESSIONAL CONDUCT

Whatever happens a nurse remains a nurse. Bradley (1984) is wrong when he suggests that the nurse abandons the nurse–patient relationship once she is attacked. Generally she has a number of duties.

(a) To make sure that she has the skills to carry out the tasks which she undertakes. She has to be competent.
(b) She must have the skills to deliver her care to a broad range of patients some of whom may become violent.
(c) While she does have the right and the duty to use reasonable force as described above she must also act in a way which does not cause unnecessary hazard to the patient.
(d) She must also return to a more normal professional nurse–patient relationship as soon as is possible.

HEALTH AND SAFETY

In addition to the above the nurse has to take account of the Health and Safety at Work Act (Jones 1982). This has two main effects. Under this act it is incumbent on an employer to make sure that methods of work are safe, that the workplace is a safe place to be and to work and that staff are instructed and trained to a level which ensures their safety. The employer should actively make sure that there are no hazards to the health and safety of employees or the public.

It is also a responsibility of the employee to report any such hazards to their employer. Any failure to act to reduce hazards at work is therefore against the law under this act. The act does not specifically mention aggression or violence but this is covered by the general duties placed upon the employer (and therefore the employee) under this act.

The TUC make a number of recommendations concerning violence and the act (TUC 1989) and this ought to be read by all nurses and their managers. Their advice is generally sound and ought to be considered when preparing policy and procedure documents which cover aggression and violence. The one criticism which can be made of their chapter covering this topic is that it fails to emphasize the employee's responsibility.

In the late 1970s an officer from the Health and Safety Executive visited a large psychiatric hospital in the north-east of England. He noted that many wards had only one nurse on duty at night and his recommendations produced the following action in the hospital. Wherever there were acutely ill male patients there had to be two male staff on duty – one of whom had to be qualified. Wherever there were acute female patients there had to be two staff on duty – one of whom had to be qualified and at least one of whom had to be female. On mixed acute wards there had to be two male and one female staff one of whom had to be qualified. This general principle should apply to all contact with the potentially violent.

An A&E department ought to have a similar mix of staff as part of its minimum staffing. Any employer who does not make this provision is most probably failing in their duty under the Health and Safety Act. Any employee who is aware of the risk and the possible solution and who does not report this to her employer is also failing in her duty under the act.

What must be emphasized again is that inaction can be as much a failure as the wrong action. Very often someone who acts in good faith but gets it wrong will be in a better legal and moral position than someone who did nothing. In my opinion the greatest failing in so many nurses is that they do not use their initiative and regularly fail to intervene in situations which need their skills.

There are courses available teaching the Home Office developed C&R techniques. Employers have a duty to send employees on these courses where there is any danger from violence or any need to confront individuals in the workplace and perhaps to and from the workplace. C&R techniques (Needham 1987) must become the norm when using physical force as a part of managing violence and aggression.

CONTRACTUAL DUTY

In addition to her professional responsibility the nurse also has a contractual duty to her employer. When she agreed to work for her employer and when her employer agreed to give her a post they jointly agreed certain things. Her employer has agreed to do such things as pay her, provide certain conditions of employment, and so on. The employee agreed to carry out certain functions often within certain criteria.

Contractual obligations tend to be less flexible than professional obligations. This gives the individual nurse less initiative but at the same time perhaps makes fewer demands on her. Most employees would seem to view the contractual obligations as being the more important. Most professional nurses would regard the professional obligation as being the primary one.

Where there is a conflict between her employer's need and her patient's need the nurse might like to consider the situation like this. She has a legal contract with her employer, and if she breaks it she can be disciplined, even dismissed. But similarly she might take the view that she has a contract with her profession and should she break that contract she can be dismissed from the profession. All nurses must be aware of the Code of Professional Conduct (UKCC 1984) but in this case items 4, 7, 10 and 11 are specially relevant.

If nursing is to develop as a profession nurses must begin to place their professional role above that of their role as employee. Only in such a position can they maximize their service to the patients. Only as a profession of autonomous practitioners can nurses effectively manage all patients in their care. Being able to exercise her skills as she sees fit is part of the effective management of the aggressive and violent patient.

SUMMARY

The nurse has a number of duties. These are prescribed by the law of the land (Health and Safety Act; Criminal Law Act), the professional bodies and by her contract with her employer. These duties may at times be in conflict. The nurse should strive to prepare herself to manage aggressive behaviour. Her priorities should include self-preservation. She has the duty and the right to use reasonable force to restrain a patient (or any other person) who is or intends to commit a crime. Reasonable force is the minimum necessary.

References

Adams, J. L. (1987) *Conceptual Blockbusting: A Guide to Better Ideas*, Penguin.

Archer, J. and Westeman, K. (1981) 'Sex differences in the aggressive behaviour of schoolchildren', *British Journal of Social Psychology*, vol. 20, pp. 31–6.

Argyle, M. (1972) *The Psychology of Interpersonal Behaviour*, Penguin.

—— (1981) *Social Skills and Health Care*, Methuen.

Asch, S. E. (1952) *Social Psychology*, Prentice Hall.

Atkinson, R. L., Atkinson, C. A. and Hilgard, E. R. (1983) *Introduction to Psychology*, 8th edition, Harcourt Brace Jovanovich.

Audley, R. J. (1967) 'What makes up a mind?', in F. G. Castles *et al.*, *Decisions, Organisations and Society*, Penguin.

Bandura, A. (1977) *Social Learning Theory*, Prentice Hall.

Barker, P. J. and Frazer, P. (1985) *The Nurse as Therapist: A Behavioural Model*, Croom Helm.

Bee, H. (1989) *The Developing Child*, Harper and Row.

Berne, E. (1966) *Games People Play*, André Deutch.

Bond, M. (1987) *Stress and Self-awareness: A Guide for Nurses*, Heinemann.

Bowlby, J. (1984) *Attachment and Loss*: vol. 1, *Attachment*; vol. 2, *Loss*, Pelican.

Bradley, D. (1984) *Accident and Emergency Nursing*, Baillière Tindall.

Brown, D. and Pedder, J. (1975) *Introduction to Psychotherapy*, Heinemann.

Bryan, J.M. and Test, M.A. (1967) 'Models and helping: naturalistic studies in aiding behaviour', *Journal of Personality and Social Psychology*, vol. 6, pp. 400–707.

Buckroyd, J. (1987) 'The nurse as counsellor', *Nursing Times*, 15 July.

Burnard, P. (1985) *Learning Human Skills: A Guide for Nurses*, Heinemann.

Burnard, P. (1986) 'Integrated self-awareness training: a holistic model', *Nurse Education Today*, vol. 6, pp. 219–22.

Burnard, P. (1989) 'Fads and fashion', *Nursing Times*, 22 February.

Butler-Sloss (1988) *Report of the Inquiry into Child Abuse in Cleveland 1987*, HMSO.

Collister, B. (1988) *Psychiatric Nursing. Person to Person*, Edward Arnold.

Cox, C. (1983) *Sociology: An Introduction for Nurses, Midwives and Health Visitors*, Butterworth.

Davis, B. (1981) 'Social skills in nursing', in Argyle (1981).

Dexter, G. and Wash, M. (1986) *Psychiatric Nursing Skills: A Patient Centred Approach*, Croom Helm.

DHSS (1975) *Regional Secure Units Design Guidelines*, HMSO.

—— (1989) *Report of the DHSS Advisory Committee on Violence to Staff (Violence to Staff)*, HMSO.

—— (Northern Ireland) (1980) *Report of the Advisory Group on the Management of Violent or Potentially Violent Patients*, HMSO.

DSS (Standing Nursing and Midwives Advisory Committee for Secretary of State for DSS and Secretary of State for Wales) (1988) *Child Protection: Guidelines for Senior Nurses and Midwives*, HMSO.

Dunn, M. (1989) 'Are you sitting comfortably?', *Nursing Times*, 9 March, pp. 29–30.

Egan, G. (1985) *The Skilled Helper: A Systematic Approach to Effective Helping*, Brooks/Cole.

ENB and WNB (1982) *Syllabus of Training 1982. Professional Register – Part 3*, ENB and WNB.

French, P. (1983) *Social Skills for Nursing Practice*, Croom Helm.

Fretwell, J. E. (1982) *Ward Teaching and Learning*, RCN.

Fries, J. F. and Crapo, L. M. (1981) *Vitality and Ageing*, Freeman.

Frost, S. and Nunkoosing, K. (1989) 'Building a strong foundation', *Nursing Times*, 1 January.

Geer, J. and Maisel, E. (1972) 'Evaluating the effects of the prediction-control confound', *Journal of Personality and Social Psychology*, vol. 23, pp. 314–19.

Guildford, J. P. (1970) 'Triads of creativity', in Vernon (1970).

Haddad, F. (1985) 'Is she fit to have a child?', *MIMS Magazine*, 15 March, p. 15.

Hamilton, J. R. and Freeman, H. (1982) *Dangerousness: Psychiatric Assessment and Management*, Gaskell.

Hammill, K. (1987) 'Seclusion: inside looking out', *Nursing Times*, 4 February, pp. 38–9.

Hardy, R. H. (1985) *Accident and Emergencies: A Practical Handbook for Personal Use*, 4th edition, Oxford Medical Publications, pp. 160–1.

Hargie, O. (ed.) (1986) *A Handbook of Communication Skills*, Croom Helm.

Hargie, O. and McCarten, P. J. (1986) *Social Skills Training and Psychiatric Nursing*, Croom Helm.

Harlow, H. F. (1971) *Learning to Love*, Albion.

Harrigan, J. A. and Steffan, J. J. (1983) 'Gaze as a turn exchange signal in group conversation', *British Journal of Social Psychology*, vol. 22, pp. 167–8.

Harris, L. (1988) 'Breaking bad news', *Nursing Times Community Outlook*, July.

Hayward, J. (1975) *Information: A Prescription Against Pain*, RCN.

Hempel, S. (1988) 'No place to lose a loved one', *Nursing Times*, 31 August.

Jones, J. A. (1983) 'Where angels fear to tread. Nursing and the concept of creativity', *Journal of Advanced Nursing*, vol. 8, pp. 405–11.

Jones, R. (1982) 'Contending with violence on the wards', *Nursing Mirror*, 23 June.

Jones, R. M. (1985) *Mental Health Act Manual*, Sweet and Maxwell.

Kabosa, A. S. C., Kahn, S. and Maddi, S. R. (1982) 'Hardiness and health: a prospective study', *Journal of Personality and Social Psychology*, vol. 42, pp. 168–77.

Kemp, R. S. and Kemp, C. H. (1978) *Child Abuse*, Fontana/Open Books.

Legge, D. and Barber, P. (1976) *Information and Skill*, Methuen.

Leopoldt, H. (1985) 'A secure and secluded spot', *Nursing Times*, 6 February, pp. 26–7.

McFarlane, J. (1976) 'The science and art of nursing', *Nursing Mirror*, 24 June, pp. 64–6.

McGregor, D. (1960) *The Human Side of Enterprise*, McGraw Hill.

Marriner, A. (1980) *Guide to Nursing Management*, C. V. Mosby.

Milgram, S. (1974) *Obedience to Authority*, Tavistock.

Milne, D., Walker, J. and Bentinck, W. (1985) 'The value of feedback', *Nursing Times*, 20 February, pp. 34–7.

MIND (1974) *Guidelines for the Care of Patients Who Exhibit Violent Behaviour in Mental and Mental Subnormality Hospitals: A Consultative Document*, MIND.

Moran, J. (1984) 'Response and responsibility', *Nursing Times*, 4 April, pp. 28–31.

Morris, D. and Marsh, P. (1988) *Tribes*, Pyramid.

Morrison, P. and le Roux, B. (1987) 'The practice of seclusion', *Nursing Times*, 13

May, pp. 62–6.

Mussen, P. M., Conger, J. J. and Kagen, J. (1969) *Child Development and Personality*, Harper and Row.

Needham, G. (1987) 'Are You Safe?', *Nursing Times*, 1 July.

Niven, N. (1989) *Health Psychology*, Churchill Livingstone.

Nurse, G. (1975) *Counselling and the Nurse*, HM&M.

Orton, H. D. (1981) *Ward Learning Climate*, RCN.

Parnes, S. J. (1970) 'Education and creativity', in Vernon (1970).

Pope, B. (1986) *Social Skills Training for Psychiatric Nurses*, Lippincott.

Priest, R. and Woolfson, G. (1978) *Minski's Handbook of Psychiatry*, Heinemann.

Rack, P. (1982) *Race, Culture and Mental Disorder*, Tavistock.

Raphael, W. Y. and Handeville, J. (1977) *Being an Outpatient*, Kings Fund.

RCN (1978) *Counselling in Nursing*, RCN.

RCN (1987) *Guidelines for Dealing with Aggression in the Accident and Emergency Department*, RCN.

RCP and RCN (1986) *Principles of Good Medical and Nursing Practice in the Management of Acts of Violence*, RCP and RCN.

Reazik, T. A. (1970) 'Psychometric measurements of creativity', in Vernon (1970).

Roper, N., Logan, W. and Tierney, A. (1983) *Using a Model of Nursing*, Churchill Livingstone.

Royal Commission on the National Health Service (1978) *Patients' Attitudes to the Hospital Service*, HMSO.

Rutter, D. R., Stephenson, G. M. and Dewey, M. E. (1981) 'Visual communication and the content and style of conversation', *British Journal of Social Psychology*, vol. 20, pp. 41–52.

Sadler, C. (1988) '3.5 million days are lost each year waiting in outpatients' departments. What can the nurses do about it?', *Nursing Times*, 3 March.

Seligman, M., Abramson, L. V., Semmel, A. and von Baeyer, C. (1979) 'Depressive attributional style', *Journal of Abnormal Psychology*, vol. 88, pp. 242–7.

Seligman, M. (1975) *Helplessness*, Freeman.

Shepherd, J. W. and Deregowski, J. B. (1981) 'Races and faces: a comparison of the responses of Africans and Europeans to faces of the same and different races', *British Journal of Social Psychology*, vol. 20, pp. 125–33.

South Birmingham Health Authority (1974a) *Guidelines for the Management of Violent Patients*, South Birmingham Health Authority.

—— (1974b) *Guidelines for the Management of Violent Patients for Nurses in Training*, Birmingham South Health Authority.

Stratton, G. M. (1897) 'Vision Without Inversion of the Retinal Image', *Psychological Review*, vol. 4, pp. 341–6.

TUC (1989) *Hazards at Work: TUC Guide to Health and Safety*, TUC.

UKCC (1984) *Code of Professional Conduct*.

Unidentified (1989) 'Only if the face fits', *Nursing Times*, 11 January.

van Larwick (1974) *In the Shadow of Man*, Fontana.

Verbal report (1983) A SWTRHA solicitor at a 1983 MHA training day.

Vernon, P. E. (1970) *Creativity*, Penguin.

Walsh, M. (1986) 'On the front line', *Nursing Times*, 10 September, pp. 55–6.

Wood, C. (1988) 'Typecasting. Is disease linked with personality?', *Nursing Times*, 30 November.

Yarbus, D. (1967) *Eye Movement and Vision*, Plenum.

Glossary

adult: one of the three positions that an individual can adopt when interacting (see **child** and **parent**). It is the reasonable and objective part of personality most effective in managing aggression.

advocacy: the idea that the nurse must act and speak on the patient's behalf when he is unable to.

affect: one of the three psychological domains. Includes such aspects as attitudes, values and emotions.

aggression: the expression of anger with an implication of violence. Aggression is normally present in all people as a potential force for action if circumstances appear to require it.

analytical therapy: a psychological therapy (usually **Freudian**) which aims to solve the patient's psychological problems through revealing and analysing the background to those problems.

assertiveness: a style of behaviour marked by clear and calm expression of ideas, feelings and needs. It is differentiated from **aggression**, **manipulation**, **passivity** and **withdrawal**.

assertion training: a therapeutic or developmental process using mostly behavioural techniques to help the individual become more assertive.

attitudes: a preset strategy for dealing with a particular event or object in the world.

authoritarian: a particular way of dealing with the world characterized by a tendency to exercise strict authority over those perceived to be lower down the hierarchy and obedience to those perceived as being superior.

behaviour: any activity which can be observed by another person.

behaviourism: the scientific study of human behaviour characterized by a belief that it is observable behaviour which is important, the underlying mechanisms being irrelevant. Modern behaviourism is less rigid.

boundaries: the limits of acceptable behaviour. When clearly defined and enforced in an adult manner can be described as 'boundary setting' and is an important therapeutic concept.

child: one of the three positions that an individual can adopt when interacting (see **adult** and **parent**). It is the part which enjoys playing but can also be very demanding.

Code of Conduct: a code issued by the United Kingdom Central Council for Nurses, Midwives and Health Visitors stating a number of important principles.

cognition: one of the three psychological domains including such aspects as thinking, knowing and perceiving.

cognitive therapy: a group of therapies dealing with cognitive processes, for example, correcting an individual's misconceptions about the perceptions others have of them.

Control and Restraint: a system devised by the Home Office to enable groups of three staff to restrain a patient, to break away from an assailant and to contain a riot. The essence of it is effectiveness and safety.

convergence: a style of thinking characterized by a tendency to concentrate on one issue and one way of doing things. Sometimes called serial thinking.

counselling: a therapeutic process in which the counsellor enables the client to work through a problem without being directive.

creativity: a group of traits including **divergency** and intelligence enabling the creative person to develop newer and more novel ideas.

democratic (management style): a style of leadership characterized by an interest in and an accommodation of the views of all those involved in or affected by decision-making.

divergency: a style of thinking characterized by a tendency to see many aspects of an issue and many ways of doing things. Sometimes called holistic thinking.

duty to care: a legal obligation for an individual to take care that her acts (or omissions) do not cause harm to others.

eclecticism: the combining of different theories or parts of theories to produce an approach tailored to suit the situation.

empathy: one of the three therapeutic qualities. The ability to appreciate the feelings and position of another individual.

extroversion: a psychological trait characterized by the individual's tendency to respond more to external factors than internal.

Freud: the proposer of a theory which included the idea of non-conscious process and of specific stages of development.

genuineness: one of the three therapeutic qualities. The considered practice of being honest during interactions.

hardy personality: a group of traits resulting in the individual being more able to tolerate stress without harmful effects. The qualities are the belief that the individual has a large degree of control over her own actions, a

commitment to what she does and being able to find challenge rather than threat in difficult situations.

interaction: the process of having any dealing with another person who is able to respond.

introversion: a psychological trait characterized by the individual's tendency to respond more to internal factors than external.

IQ: a measure of the individual's intellectual ability. Much criticized, it remains a good general guide when used properly.

manipulation: the practice of using devious and dishonest means to achieve ends.

mental health: a state of mental well-being best described by Atkinson *et al.* (1983). It is included in the preferred name for most mental nurses.

modelling: the act of behaving in a particular way to demonstrate that behaviour so that another person may copy it. The process involves both conscious and non-conscious elements.

morality: part of the system of beliefs relating to the rights and wrongs of behaviour.

nature/nurture: the debate over the influences on the development of the individual. In reality it is impossible to distinguish most aspects of these.

non-verbal communication: any body movement, posture or sign which contributes to the message being sent.

objectivity: the ability to see a situation or event in an unbiased and unselfish way.

open positions: the positions which convey that the person is open to approach and is not defending themselves against interaction.

parent: one of the three positions that an individual can adopt when interacting (see **adult** and **child**). It is the part which protects and supervises others.

passivity: the failure to take any action.

personality: the total of all the individual differences occurring in a person.

prejudice: a judgement about a person, event or situation made before encountering that person, event or situation.

problem-solving: a particular form of decision-making involving four stages: assessment, planning, action and evaluation. It has been adopted by the nursing profession as the best way to make decisions about patient care.

reasonable force: the minimum force needed to prevent or stop a crime being committed or to detain the person responsible for committing a crime.

regression: the act of returning to a way of functioning associated with an earlier stage of development. This is usually at a time of stress and is usually a bad strategy.

respect: one of the three therapeutic qualities. A recognition of the individuality and value of another person.

restraint: any action by a nurse using physical means to limit the behaviour of a patient. Usually refers to the organized and intentional holding of a patient but can include mechanical and chemical restraint.

role: a set of behaviours associated with a particular social position.

role strain: conflict arising from contradictory demands made by the roles occupied by a person.

schizophrenia: a group of illnesses little understood but marked by the individual's isolation from others and an inability to separate imagination from reality. May be caused by concrete thinking.

seclusion: the act of removing and keeping a patient separated from the presence of other patients and visitors even when there are staff present.

self: all parts of the individual's being which are included in their concept of themself. A term used to differentiate the self from others.

self-awareness: an understanding of own feelings, thoughts and behaviour. A general skill which can be cultivated and used to help the individual develop. It is associated with good mental health.

sick role: a role in which the individual fulfils the expectations of someone suffering from an illness, including the desire to recover.

Skinner: American psychologist who championed the ideas of behaviourism. Seen by many as an extremist although he has made a valuable contribution to the understanding of behaviour.

social skills: described here as any skilled activity which contributes to the individual's social functioning. Seen by others as more specifically associated with communication and interaction.

subjectivity: the process of seeing something only from a selfish point of view, thus being biased and possibly unrealistic.

traits: the separate qualities of the individual which when combined contribute to personality. The study of traits gives more reliable information than the study of types.

Transactional Analysis: the study of interactions according to the ideas of Berne. Used in a modified way here to discuss interactions.

violence: any physical act against others, self or property which is intended to cause damage.

withdrawal: the act of refusing to interact.

Index